D0363201

HIGH BLOOD PRESSURE

Dr Eoin O'Brien and Professor Kevin O'Malley are co-directors of the Blood Pressure Clinic at the Charitable Infirmary, one of Dublin's major teaching hospitals, and have many years of experience in treating patients with high blood pressure.

Dr O'Brien is also Consultant Cardiologist at the Infirmary, and a frequent contributor to medical journals. As a member of the Council of the Irish Heart Foundation, he is closely involved in health education.

Professor O'Malley is Professor of Clinical Pharmacology, Royal College of Surgeons in Ireland, and Consultant Physician at the Charitable Infirmary and St Laurence Hospital, Dublin. He has written over 100 scientific papers on high blood pressure and the study of drugs in man.

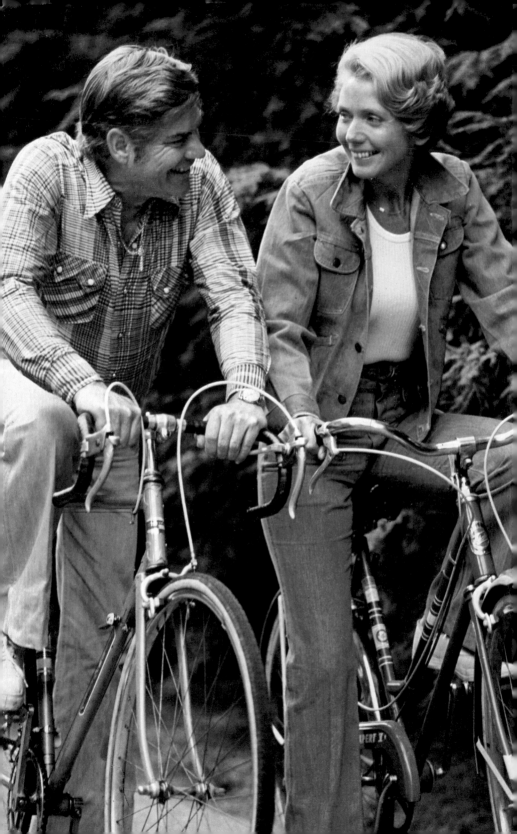

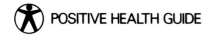 POSITIVE HEALTH GUIDE

HIGH BLOOD PRESSURE

What it means for you,
and how to control it

Dr Eoin O'Brien
FRCP, MRCP

and

Professor Kevin O'Malley
MD, PhD, FRCP

Foreword by Dr Walter Somerville
Recently President of the British Cardiac Society

MARTIN DUNITZ

Reprinted 1983

First published in the United Kingdom in 1982
by Martin Dunitz Limited, London

British Library Cataloguing in
Publication Data
O'Brien, Eoin
    High blood pressure. – (Positive health guides)
    1. Hypertension
    I. Title   II. O'Malley, Kevin   III. Series
    616.1'32   RC685.H8

    ISBN 0-906348-23-4
    ISBN 0-906348-24-2 Pbk

Phototypeset in Garamond by Bookens, Saffron Walden, Essex

Printed in Singapore by Koon Wah Printing Pte. Ltd.

CONTENTS

FOREWORD

Walter Somerville, CBE, MD, FRCP, FACC
Recently President of the British Cardiac Society

The attack on high blood pressure intensifies every year. Conferences, symposia and textbooks proliferate and even though cynics mutter among themselves that more problems are created than solved, some progress can claim to have been made. Early diagnosis is the most promising tactic, but since high blood pressure develops silently and without warning, how to detect it in its early stages remains an unsolved problem. An attractive approach, and the one most likely to succeed, centres on the perceptive public demand for information on how the heart works and what makes blood pressure rise. The main obstacle in meeting this demand is the innate inability of most experts to communicate what they know. Academics writing for the public often treat their readers as morons or blind them with scientific gobbledegook. It is time that the layman who complains that the workings of his body are wrapped in the secrecy of medical jargon should be listened to . . . .

His pleas have now been heard by Dr O'Brien and Professor O'Malley. Well informed and distinguished in the field of high blood pressure, they have the talent of communicating without pomposity or self-consciousness. The gist of their message is that high blood pressure and its problems cannot be solved by the doctors alone; the layman must take some responsibility for prevention and a great deal for management and control. They dispel the mystique from home blood-pressure measurement, discount the dangers of a little learning, and are committed to the value of knowledge. They know the many pitfalls surrounding high-blood-pressure management, the disabling side-effects of treatment, and the risk of creating a race of neurotics devoting their lives to measuring their blood pressure and cholesterol. Yet they avoid the most perilous pitfall of evangelistic zeal, the surest way of defeating the entire prevention movement. The layman may take up this book with my assurance that it is sensibly written, won't turn him into a neurotic and may in time rescue him from premature disease and disability.

INTRODUCTION

If you have high blood pressure you can still lead a normal active life. You can go on playing squash or golf. You won't have to give up gardening or any other activity provided you are otherwise fit. Indeed, your doctor may even encourage you to take more exercise. High blood pressure does not of itself make you feel unwell and only rarely does it cause symptoms. Why then need we bother about it?

A small rise in blood pressure is not necessarily harmful, but prolonged elevation of blood pressure over a number of years greatly increases the risk of diseases of the heart and circulation such as stroke and heart attack. If untreated, high blood pressure can cause many serious problems, and it can also shorten life. In this book we want to show beyond all doubt how important a risk to health it is. We believe that if we were all fully aware of the implications of raised blood pressure, we would make sure that our blood pressure was checked regularly.

There is, in fact, only one way to know for sure whether you have high blood pressure, and that is by having it measured with an instrument known as a sphygmomanometer. Fortunately, this can be done simply and accurately by any trained person such as a doctor or nurse, and more recently by lay people. Because we feel that being able to measure your blood pressure at home is helpful to both you and your doctor, considerable emphasis is given in chapter three to the correct use of the sphygmomanometer.

Once high blood pressure has been diagnosed, only your doctor can decide what kind of treatment, if any, you need. Not everyone with high blood pressure needs drug treatment. Many other factors may be important such as smoking, your diet and activity, so lifestyle changes like giving up smoking, losing weight and taking exercise could also help to bring down your blood pressure levels. In some cases they may be sufficient.

During the last twenty years there have been considerable advances in pharmacological research, and new and effective drugs for lowering high blood pressure are now available. But all drugs, however simple, have some unwanted side-effects, and this holds true of drugs that lower blood pressure. There is great individual variation in response to drugs and it may take a little while for you and your doctor to find the most suitable drug for you.

We believe that it is very important for people with high blood pressure to know something about the drugs they are taking, and particularly about any possible side-effects, so that they can discuss them with their doctor. Experience has shown us that drugs prescribed for high blood pressure are all too often not taken according to instructions. This is in fact a major problem in the control of high blood pressure, and in writing this book we hope to show how the successful control of high blood pressure depends on close co-operation between you and your doctor. Understanding what high blood pressure is all about will, we trust, help to improve this vital relationship.

1 THE PROBLEM OF HIGH BLOOD PRESSURE

How common is it?

High blood pressure is a world-wide condition of epidemic proportions. For most doctors it is the single most common chronic disorder encountered in practice. It has been estimated that in Western countries somewhere between 15 and 20 per cent of the adult population have high blood pressure. Blood pressure usually rises with age and a blood pressure which would be considered abnormally high in a ten-year-old would be quite satisfactory in a seventy-year-old person.

High blood pressure is relatively rare in children, but very common in old age. Among young adults men are more likely to have it than women. With increasing age sexual equality reasserts itself and approximately 40 per cent of both men and women in the fifty-five to sixty-five age group have higher than normal pressure.

High blood pressure during pregnancy is a special problem and will be discussed in chapter nine which looks at the whole question of women and high blood pressure. However, it can be said here that if you have not previously had high blood pressure but develop it during the last few months of pregnancy the chances are that pressure will return to normal after the baby is born.

How do you know if you have high blood pressure?

Approximately 60 per cent of those with high blood pressure are unaware that they have it. For most people with high blood pressure there are no tell-tale symptoms. In fact, the majority of people with this condition have no symptoms whatsoever. This means, therefore, that high blood pressure is usually diagnosed by chance, for instance at a routine physical check-up requested by an insurance company or new employer. Or your doctor may take the opportunity to measure your blood pressure when you happen to be in his surgery on a quite unrelated matter, such as a cold or backache.

If on such a visit your doctor overlooks the blood-pressure check, tell him you would like to know what your blood pressure is. It will only take a minute or two to measure it. Make a note of his answer as it may be useful to have this information in the future. If your pressure is normal your doctor will probably say that you can wait another twelve months or more before you need to have another check. On the other hand, if your pressure is higher than normal you should listen carefully to his advice and ask about anything that you don't fully understand.

What does it mean?

One of the first things to get clear is what is meant by the words high blood pressure or hypertension, as it is also called. You may hear your doctor use this word and it is as well to know that both terms mean the same and can be used synonymously. We feel it is better not to use the term hypertension because it tends to suggest an association with stress or tension. In this book, therefore, we have preferred to keep to the words high blood pressure.

There are two components of blood pressure: when the heart is contracting the pressure is highest, and when the heart is relaxing the pressure is at its low point. The unit of measurement used internationally in blood pressure measurement is the millimetre of mercury (mmHg). If your doctor tells you that your blood pressure reading is, say, 160 over 110, he will probably write this down as 160/110 mmHg. He may also take a reading when you are lying down since blood pressure varies according to whether you are sitting, standing, lying or have just indulged in strenuous exercise. It also varies from person to person so it is hard to define normal blood pressure, but see the next chapter for a fuller discussion.

The importance of finding out

The small but significant number of untreated people who arrive in the doctor's surgery already suffering from one or other of the serious complications of high blood pressure shows that there is a great need for early detection. Many cases of stroke occur in people whose high blood pressure has never been treated effectively and sometimes they have never even had their blood pressure measured. Similarly, most doctors know of patients whose heart attacks or kidney failure might well have been avoided if they had had treatment for their high blood pressure.

A major stroke can kill or it can leave a person severely incapacitated and unable to cope on his or her own. The family will suffer as the patient becomes dependent on relatives and it is all too easy to visualize the economic consequences of the breadwinner becoming unemployable at, say, fifty years of age.

What should you do?

If you have never had your blood pressure checked it is obviously a good idea to ask your doctor to check it on your next visit. Or you can use one of the public machines if one is available near you.

A number of symptoms are sometimes associated with high blood pressure but, as we have said, high blood pressure itself rarely causes symptoms. If you suffer from headache, dizziness, fatigue or nosebleed, it does not therefore mean that you have high blood pressure. You should report them to your doctor and he may then check your pressure, but these are all symptoms that in fact occur almost just as frequently in people with normal blood pressure.

Let us assume, however, that although you feel fit and healthy your doctor has found a high reading. One of the first things you will want to know is what exactly is high blood pressure? In the next chapter we shall try to answer this question.

2 WHAT IS HIGH BLOOD PRESSURE?

Blood pressure and the circulation

Before you can understand *high* blood pressure it is necessary to appreciate what blood pressure itself is. This in turn requires an explanation of how the blood flows through the body – that is, the circulation. The circulation (or cardiovascular system) consists of a pump, the heart, and two circuits around which the blood travels. In one circuit, known as the pulmonary circulation, the blood which has returned to the heart is pumped through the lungs where it takes up oxygen. The blood then returns to the heart and is pumped to the rest of the body. This is the second circuit, known to doctors as the systemic circulation.

The proper functioning of this system depends on three main factors. First, the pump (the heart) must be in working order so that blood is pumped around the circuits. Second, the blood vessels must be in good condition so that they can carry the blood to every part of the body. Third, there must be sufficient pressure in the system for it to work efficiently. This pressure – the blood pressure – is the force exerted by the blood pumped from the heart against the walls of the arteries. Or, to put it another way, blood pressure is the amount of force required to circulate the blood round the body.

How the circulation works
Initially the blood goes along the aorta, which is the large blood vessel leading from the heart. The arteries branch at various points from the aorta and carry blood vessels to the head, limbs and organs, in fact to every part of the body. The blood vessels divide several times into smaller and smaller blood vessels – the capillaries. The capillaries have very thin walls across which oxygen, carbon dioxide, nutrients and waste products can be passed to and from the blood and body fluids. The capillaries link with the veins. These are the blood vessels responsible for collecting the blood and returning it to the heart, where the

cycle starts once more.

The circulatory system is a closed one. Strategically placed valves on each side of the heart ensure that the blood flows in the correct direction. In order to maintain the circulation everybody must have a certain level of blood pressure.

What is normal blood pressure?

Blood pressure is kept within certain limits by the interaction of many factors, but basically by the pumping action of the heart and the width of the blood vessels. If for any reason the pumping action of the heart gets faster or the resistance offered by the blood vessels increases, blood pressure tends to rise. During the course of an ordinary day your blood pressure is constantly changing. Strenuous exercise tends to make the pressure go up, as does stress. If you lie down or rest, your pressure will go down. This is all quite normal. It is only when blood pressure rises markedly and remains high that a person can be said to have high blood pressure.

It must be emphasized that there is no clearly defined blood pressure level above which pressure is too high and below which pressure is normal. In fact, when blood pressure is measured in large groups of people we find that the readings are distributed over a wide range so that some people have quite low readings and others very high, but most people have levels between these extremes.

With each heartbeat your blood pressure undergoes a pattern of change. The highest pressure occurs shortly after the blood is pumped from the heart into the large blood vessels and this peak pressure is known as the systolic pressure (see diagram on page 35).The lower or trough pressure is referred to as the diastolic pressure and this occurs when the heart is relaxed and being filled by the blood returning through the veins – preparing for another heartbeat.

Fortunately, we can measure systolic and diastolic pressure reasonably accurately without having to gain direct access to the blood vessel, by using an instrument called the sphygmomanometer. This consists of a cuff which is placed around your upper arm. The cuff is connected to a small rubber pump and to a mercury column. When the cuff is inflated with the pump the pressure of the cuff increases until it is sufficient to stop your artery pulsating. Then the pressure is slowly released by means of a valve; and by listening with a stethoscope over the artery for certain changes of sound in the returning blood flow the doctor can read off from the mercury column your systolic and diastolic pressures. The exact method of measuring blood pressure is described in detail in chapter three.

Despite the reservations we have about using a precise dividing line between normal blood pressure and high blood pressure, it is necessary to use some such arbitrary values. The World Health Organization has defined normal blood pressure as a systolic pressure equal to or less than 140 mmHg together with a diastolic value equal to or less than 90 mmHg.

What counts as high blood pressure?

High blood pressure has been defined by the same organization as a sustained systolic pressure equal to or greater than 160 mmHg and/or diastolic values equal to or greater than 95

Most people have systolic blood pressure of between 100 and 160 mmHg, but some have values outside these limits.

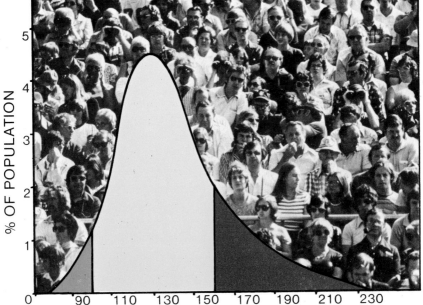

Distribution of blood pressure levels over the population

mmHg. The term borderline is used for those with blood pressure values between normal and high.

In high blood pressure the systolic and diastolic pressures tend to rise together, but this is not invariably so. Some people, particularly the elderly, have a much greater increase in the systolic than the diastolic pressure. In such cases the diastolic pressure may be normal or near normal.

Sometimes the severity of high blood pressure is graded according to the diastolic value alone. Mild blood pressure is considered to be a diastolic pressure between 95 and 104 mmHg, moderate is 105 to 114, and severe is any value above this. These are only rough divisions, however. Most people with high blood pressure belong to the mild group. (There is still a lot of controversy as to whether all people in this group should be given drug treatment.)

Another way to define high blood pressure is to relate blood pressure values with other problems linked to high blood pressure. In 1959 the insurance companies in the United States published their experiences with blood pressure compared to life expectancy. They showed that people with the highest pressures had the shortest life expectancy, premature death being related to diseases of the heart, stroke and kidney disease. Those with low blood pressure values had the best chances, while people with mild blood pressure were somewhere between the two.

The late Sir George Pickering, who was a world-renowned expert on this subject defined high blood pressure as that blood pressure which is better treated than left alone.

How does the body control blood pressure?

Like all physiological systems the circulation is maintained by complicated control mechanisms. Minute-to-minute control of blood pressure is mediated through special sensors in the large blood vessels. These sensors are called the baroreceptors. They are capable of detecting tiny changes in blood pressure. When blood pressure falls there is a reflex which increases the heart rate and constricts the blood vessels, so that the pressure returns to its earlier level. But if you have high blood pressure, the sensitivity of the baroreceptors is altered so that higher pressures do not have this effect. The circulation seems to have become accustomed to operating at a higher pressure.

Renin
Another important mechanism in the body for maintaining blood pressure is the renin system. A change in blood pressure, let us say a reduction, causes a release of renin from the kidneys. Renin is an enzyme that is responsible for the formation of a very potent substance called angiotensin that constricts the blood vessels. When the vessels contract, resistance in the circulation increases and so the pressure rises.

Angiotensin also has a second action: it increases the release from the adrenal gland of the hormone aldosterone which controls the amount of salt and water excreted by the kidneys. More salt and water is then retained, which, in turn, increases the volume of fluid in the circulation. This increases pressure. In some people with high blood pressure it does seem that the renin system is overactive. These people have high levels of renin in their bodies and respond better to drugs which lower renin release.

Adrenaline (epinephrine)
Another hormone involved in the control of blood pressure is adrenaline (called epinephrine in North America) and its close relative noradrenaline (called norepinephrine). The amount of these hormones available to exert their effect is determined by the nervous system. It has been suggested that in many patients with high blood pressure there is an increased level of these substances, but this has never been completely proved, except in one specific and very rare disorder.

The kidney
The kidney has a central role in blood pressure regulation because it is the source of renin, the site of action of aldosterone and it handles the body's salt. (Salt has a very controversial role in high blood pressure, and will be discussed in chapter four.) One theory about the cause of high blood pressure says that a defect in salt handling by the kidney is a major factor. According to this theory, the kidney fails to eliminate as much salt as it should so the blood volume, and with it blood pressure, increases.

What problems can high blood pressure cause?

Many people believe that high blood pressure causes headache, dizzy spells and nosebleeds. These symptoms may occur if you have high blood pressure, but they are in fact unusual. Furthermore, as we have said, they may also occur just as frequently in people with normal blood pressure.

Hardening of the arteries
The blood vessels take the brunt of high blood pressure, notably those in the brain, kidneys and heart. The increased pressure leads to thickening and twisting of the blood vessels. There is disruption of the smooth inner lining of the vessels and these become irregular and block the flow of blood. Thus, high blood pressure accelerates the process of arterial hardening and narrowing known as atherosclerosis.

In these abnormal vessels there is then an increased tendency to thrombosis, or clot formation. In the heart this can lead to blockage of the coronary blood vessels resulting in a heart attack; in the brain, blockage of a blood vessel leads to paralysis and speech disturbances – known as stroke. Alternatively, bleeding can occur because of the high pressure in the damaged and weakened brain blood vessels and again this can lead to a stroke because the brain tissues are destroyed.

Heart trouble
High blood pressure contributes to the development of coronary artery disease, the commonest form of heart disease in Western society. The increase in pressure puts an extra load on the heart. As we have seen earlier the heart can cope to a certain extent, but when blood pressure elevation is moderate to severe the heart may compensate by becoming enlarged. In prolonged and severe untreated high blood pressure, the heart may not be able to function adequately. This is known as heart failure, which causes shortness of breath during physical exertion. The heart does not stop altogether; what happens is that it fails to supply adequate amounts of blood to all parts of the body.

Kidney problems
Long-standing and severe high blood pressure may also lead to changes in the blood vessels of the kidney. Again the hallmark is

thickening of the vessels and this may lead to a reduction in the flow of blood to the kidney with subsequent deterioration of its function. As with the heart, the kidney does not cease working – it simply is not as efficient as it should be.

Effect on the eye

The eye is the only part of the body that we can look directly into to observe its blood vessels. To do this doctors use an instrument called an ophthalmoscope. In high blood pressure there may be some thickening and increased twisting of these blood vessels which can be observed with this instrument. In really severe high blood pressure these blood vessels may leak blood cells and plasma (plasma is the colourless fluid part of the blood which contains the cells) and these can also be seen on examination. For the vast majority of people with high blood pressure eyesight is not affected.

Does high blood pressure lower life expectancy?

The short answer is yes. People with untreated high blood pressure cannot expect to live as long as those with normal blood pressure, but of course the effect on life expectancy depends on the severity of the high blood pressure and on a number of other factors.

The true significance of the complications of high blood pressure are brought home when we look at the statistics of death and illness related to the condition. High blood pressure is a major contributor to stroke, and heart and kidney disease, which together are responsible for more deaths than any other disease, including cancer.

The largest current population study of high blood pressure is at Framingham in Massachusetts. Dr William Kannel, a director of the Framingham Study, has found that people with high blood pressure are four times as likely to have heart failure and have three times as many heart attacks and seven times as many strokes as their counterparts with normal blood pressure.

It is little wonder that the insurance companies see blood pressure as an important factor in assessing the life expectancy of their potential clients. Premiums are fixed with this factor in mind. An example may help. A forty-five-year-old man with a

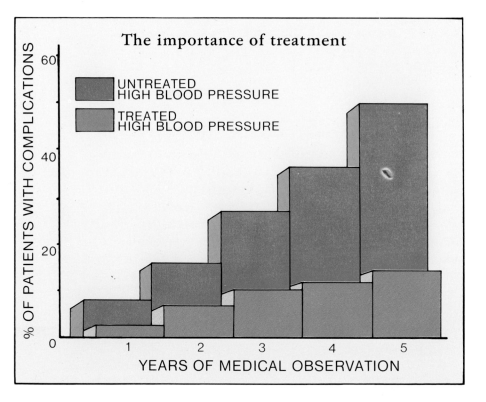

The importance of treatment

UNTREATED
HIGH BLOOD PRESSURE

TREATED
HIGH BLOOD PRESSURE

% OF PATIENTS WITH COMPLICATIONS

YEARS OF MEDICAL OBSERVATION

Untreated high blood pressure can lead to stroke, heart attacks and kidney disease. When treated, the risk of these complications is significantly reduced.

systolic pressure of 120 and a diastolic level of 80 mmHg may expect to live to over seventy years of age. A man of much the same age with a systolic pressure of 140 and a diastolic of 95 mmHg may expect to live six years less. This is very mild high blood pressure and the greater the elevation of blood pressure the greater the reduction in life expectancy, so that for severe high blood pressure twenty years or more may be cut from the normal expectation.

However, when the condition is controlled the outlook is much brighter. Appropriate blood pressure treatment prevents the complications described above and in many cases allows normal life expectancy. But we must detect high blood pressure before we can treat it and this means there must be regular blood pressure checks.

3 MEASURING YOUR BLOOD PRESSURE

In recent years there has been a slow but steady increase particularly in North America but also in Europe in the number of people who have learnt to measure their own blood pressure. It can be measured simply and conveniently at home and provided it is done according to instructions we believe that home measurement of blood pressure is helpful to both patient and doctor. Although blood pressure was discovered a long time ago, we have only been able to measure it since the beginning of this century.

In the past

It was the Reverend Stephen Hales, a rather austere eighteenth-century English clergyman from Kent, who first actually realized what the blood pressure was. From an experiment on a horse he found that when a tube was fitted into a main artery, blood would rise in the tube more than 8ft (2.5m) above the level of the heart.

It took another hundred years before this important discovery was put to practical use. Towards the end of the nineteenth century a number of devices for the measurement of blood were invented, but it was not until 1896 that an Italian physiologist called Scipione Riva-Rocci developed the sphygmomanometer with which we are familiar today. Doctors now had for the first time a measuring machine that was portable, accurate, easy to use and did not cause discomfort to the patient.

But a further advance was needed before it became possible to measure the diastolic blood pressure accurately. During the Russo-Japanese war of 1905 a Russian surgeon, Nicolai Segeyovitch Korotkoff, became interested in injuries to blood vessels when serving in Manchuria. He discovered that if a stethoscope was placed over the main artery of the upper arm – the brachial artery – after a Riva-Rocci cuff on the arm had been inflated, no sounds were heard. If the cuff was slowly deflated sounds would be heard at the point corresponding to the appearance of the radial pulse at the wrist, that is, the systolic pressure. If you continue listening as pressure in the cuff falls the sounds develop a murmuring quality and shortly afterwards disappear.

Korotkoff realized that the point of disappearance was the diastolic pressure and his discovery together with that of Riva-Rocci gave doctors a ready and reliable means of measuring both the systolic and diastolic pressure. It is a tribute to those pioneers that the method of blood measurement used today has changed very little since their discoveries.

Let us now return to the present and look at why and how you should put this method into practice.

Why do you need to keep track of blood pressure?

Blood pressure is constantly changing. It is influenced by many emotional and environmental factors, all of which make it difficult to obtain an accurate measurement of the true blood pressure. But if, over a period of weeks or even months, blood pressure is measured regularly every day, a more complete picture emerges.

After reading this book you may want to ask your doctor if he thinks home recording would be helpful for you. Or your doctor may suggest the idea. Experience has shown that almost everyone can learn to take their own blood pressure, even without prior medical training, in a short period of time.

Keeping a record
Your doctor will tell you how often you need to measure your blood pressure. Usually twice a day – morning and evening – is sufficient, but sometimes more frequent measurements are needed. If your blood pressure is stable and satisfactory a few recordings a week may suffice. You should enter your measurements in a chart or booklet like the one illustrated overleaf, giving the date, time and place of the recording; the systolic and diastolic pressures for the morning and evening; and the dose of any drug or drugs you are taking.

Home measurement chart

BLOOD PRESSURE RECORD				MEDICATION	
DATE	PLACE	TIME	PRESSURE SYSTOLIC / DIASTOLIC	NAME & STRENGTH	No.
4·4·8¹	Home	9am.	150/95	PRESSUREX : 50 mg.	1
	Home	6pm.	160/90	" "	1
5·4·8¹	Home	9am.	140/85	" "	1
	Home	6:30pm	145/90	" "	1

If you are going to measure your own blood pressure, it will be useful to construct a recording chart along these lines.

What you will need

The two items that you will need for measuring your own blood pressure are a sphygmomanometer, which measures pressure, and a stethoscope, to listen over the artery in the arm for the sounds which indicate systolic and diastolic blood pressure.

What it will cost
It is always difficult to be specific about prices because with continuing inflation they are liable to go up from year to year, if not more often. However, having said that, we can now say that at the time of going to press a good mercury sphygmomanometer (see page 24) costs around £30 (about US $60, Australian $90). Aneroid models (see page 25) are usually cheaper. A stethoscope should not cost you more than £5 (US $10, Australian $15). In other words for the price of a medium-sized portable radio you can buy all the equipment you need.

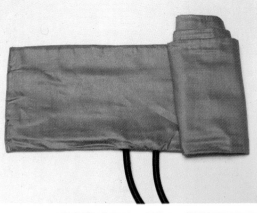

1. The sphygmomanometer cuff, inside which is the inflatable bladder. One tube leads to the measuring scale; the other to the inflation bulb. 2. The scale of a mercury sphygmomanometer, giving readings in millimetres of mercury (mmHg). 3. The bulb which is used to inflate the sphygmomanometer cuff. Above it is the circular air-release valve for deflating the cuff.

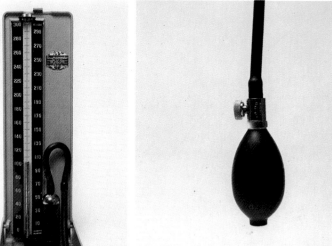

Choosing the equipment

Factors to bear in mind when choosing a sphygmomanometer for home use are: simplicity of use, cost, accuracy and reliability.

The most popular sphygmomanometers in general use today are the mercury and aneroid types. Both consist of:

1. a cuff which encircles the arm and encloses an inflatable rubber bladder;
2. a measuring scale to indicate the applied pressure;
3. an inflation bulb which allows air to be blown into the inflatable bladder;
4. a control valve which can be adjusted to deflate the pressure at any desired rate.

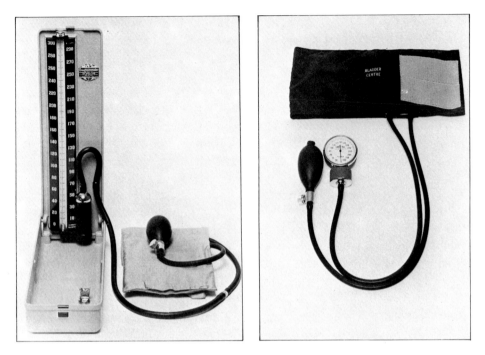

The mercury sphygmomanometer (*left*). The aneroid sphygmomanometer (*right*).

The cuff that is wrapped round the arm is made of an inelastic cloth and secured by Velcro surfaces, or by hooks. The dimensions of the inflatable rubber bladder inside the cuff should depend on the size of the arm. A bladder which is too short or too narrow will give falsely high pressures, and one which is too wide or too long will give falsely low pressures. Choose a bladder made of rubber not plastic as the latter can leak and crack after a time.

The mercury sphygmomanometer

The mercury sphygmomanometer works on the simple principle of balancing liquids with pressure. The long glass tube which forms the scale is part of a U-shaped system containing mercury; the other side of the tube is more squat, and can be seen adjoining the right-hand edge of the scale in the illustration above. When pressure is applied to this system the mercury is pushed up the scale, which gives a reading in millimetres of mercury (written as mmHg). The scale should be easy to read. The zero level of the column of mercury serves as a constant visible check on the accuracy of the instrument.

The aneroid sphygmomanometer

In aneroid instruments the pressure to be measured is applied to a bellows-like assembly of corrugated metal discs soldered or welded together to form an airtight chamber behind the measuring dial. When air pressure is applied, a stretching or expansion of the bellows occurs. This movement is transmitted and amplified by a geared linkage to drive an indicating pointer. A hairspring attached to the pointer returns the pointer downscale when pressure is released.

Semi-automated machines

There are also a number of semi-automated devices available today. A small microphone is incorporated in the cuff and placed over the main artery of the upper arm to detect the Korotkoff sounds (see page 21) which when detected give an audible or visual signal. Some of these machines provide a digital readout of the systolic and diastolic pressures. This has the advantage of dispensing with the need to use a stethoscope to listen to the sounds. However, there are some disadvantages: many of these machines are not properly assessed for accuracy, and even if accurate initially there is no guarantee that they will remain so after continued use; also, being technically more complicated, they are more liable to develop faults and they must then be returned to the manufacturer; finally, they are generally more expensive than the standard mercury machines.

Having considered the advantages and disadvantages of the three types of sphygmomanometer, our conclusions are that the simplest, the least expensive, the most reliable, the most accurate, the best tried and the most durable of them all is the mercury sphygmomanometer.

The stethoscope

There are a large variety of stethoscopes available. Many of these are cheap and of poor quality, but there is no need to go to great expense and buy a stethoscope of a better quality than you need to measure blood pressure. Choose one with good earpieces that fit snugly and firmly.

The endpiece of the stethoscope can be flat – a diaphragm endpiece – or conical – the bell endpiece. Some models have both types of endpiece. A bell endpiece gives better sound reproduction, but a diaphragm is easier to secure with the fingers of one hand and covers a larger area, so we usually

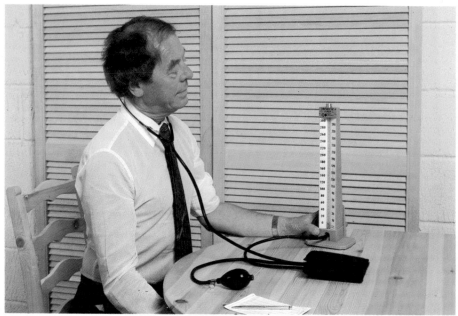

1. Placing the equipment
2. Putting on the cuff

3. Palpating the brachial artery

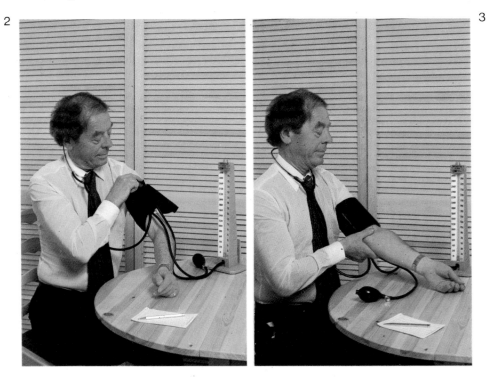

How to measure your own blood pressure

1 Place sphygmo-manometer on table. Sit beside it and place arm on table at heart level. 2 Wrap cuff around arm keeping centre of bladder over inside of arm. Secure cuff so it is not too tight or loose. It can be put on over a shirt sleeve which should not be rolled into a tight band. 3 Locate pulse of brachial artery with thumb at inside front of elbow. 4 Place stetho-scope endpiece (here inside cuff) over artery and inflate cuff to 30 mmHg above disappearance of pulse sounds. 5 Turn valve to slowly deflate cuff and listen for sound of pulse returning; the reading at this point indicates systolic pressure. Continue deflating until pulse sounds disappear; the reading at this point indicates diastolic pressure. Occasionally the sounds do not dis-appear, in which case, the point at which sounds take on a different, muffled quality indicates diastolic pressure. Record pressures to nearest 5 mmHg. Always deflate cuff completely before repeating measurement.

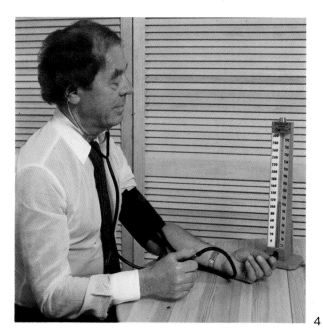

4

4. Pumping the bulb   5. Releasing the pressure and taking systolic and diastolic readings

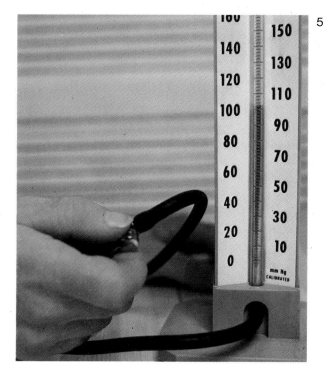

5

recommend the diaphragm type.

Sphygmomanometers specially designed for home use are now available which incorporate a stethoscope (see illustrations on pages 26 and 27). The endpiece is securely attached to the inside of the cuff leaving one hand free which otherwise would have to hold the stethoscope in place over the artery.

Sources of possible error

A major source of error is the person himself. You may be nervous or anxious; perhaps you have just had a large meal or do not feel comfortable physically. Your attention may wander or you may be in too much of a hurry.

Because of the mechanics involved, the aneroid gauge is subject to considerably more potential error than the simple mercury sphygmomanometer. The system of levers used can stick, and be affected by the jolts and knocks of everyday use.

Some aneroid gauges have an internal 'stop' so that the instrument will always register zero when pressure is not applied, which gives the user a false indication of accuracy. Better-quality gauges do not have this mechanism. But in any case, the return of the indicating pointer to the zero marking on the dial is by no means an infallible way of determining the accuracy of the instrument.

Finally there is the question of the accuracy of the sphygmomanometer itself. It may come as a surprise to you to learn that surveys of hospital sphygmomanometers have shown that nearly half of those in use on the wards are inaccurate, mainly because of inadequate maintenance. It may be an even greater surprise to hear that some sphygmomanometers being sold to the public and the medical profession have not been properly assessed for accuracy. This is especially true for many of the semi-automated devices now available. It is therefore of vital importance not only to make sure that your instrument is accurate, but also to make sure that it is regularly maintained.

How to maintain your sphygmomanometer

One of the great advantages of the mercury sphygmomanometer

is that it can be maintained by the user who can easily obtain and replace any defective parts. A yearly check should be sufficient.

It is necessary to check an aneroid gauge at least every six months. This is important because the instrument may be giving inaccurate measurements without the user being aware that anything is wrong. If you suspect that your instrument is inaccurate or if it is behaving erratically, you must take it to be serviced or return it to the manufacturer.

The following is a check list of points to watch for.

General condition   The condition of the box or case is often an indication of how well the instrument has been cared for. If your sphygmomanometer has been in use for a long time and its general condition is poor, then it may be wiser to replace it with a new instrument.

The scale   When the tube gets dirty it can be cleaned with a pipe cleaner, using first a mild detergent and then alcohol or ether.

The cuff and bladder   The fabric of the cuff should be in good condition. If the cuff is the tapering kind it should be long enough to encircle the arm several times. Velcro surfaces must be effective, and when they lose their grip they should be discarded.

Tubing, pump and control valve   All rubber parts should be kept in good condition. Cracked or perished rubber makes accurate measurement difficult. The tubing should be long enough to permit comfortable use, and connections must be airtight and easy to disconnect. The control valve is a common source of error and you should keep a spare one handy.

We believe that if you follow the guidelines suggested in this chapter you will be able to measure your blood pressure at home simply and accurately. But now let us look at the more complicated question of what causes high blood pressure.

4 WHAT CAUSES HIGH BLOOD PRESSURE?

For the vast majority of people with high blood pressure, probably more than 95 per cent, the cause of their raised pressure is not known. This does not of course mean that there is no cause, but rather that the cause or causes have not been identified. This form of high blood pressure is usually called 'essential' or 'primary' hypertension.

For a small minority of people with high blood pressure, less than 5 per cent, there is a specific, identifiable cause for their condition. The cause, or causes, can be detected by the appropriate clinical examination and by carrying out the relevant tests. These are usually done in hospital. This group of people is said to have 'secondary' high blood pressure. The term 'secondary' means that the blood pressure is raised because of some identified cause. We will first deal with the more common problem of high blood pressure that does not have a demonstrable cause.

High blood pressure with no identified cause

To simplify matters, when we use the term 'high blood pressure' in the present context we are referring to 'primary' high blood pressure.

The search for a cause or causes of high blood pressure has been the concern of medical researchers for many years. Indeed the pace of work seems to be accelerating year by year. Most investigators in the field now consider that there is probably no single factor responsible for high blood pressure. But, by examining the aspects of our environment that are known to affect blood pressure and the genetic influences at work, our understanding of high blood pressure does become a little clearer.

Heredity

When attempting to find the cause of a disease we must consider the contribution of the genetic make-up of the individual (or population) as well as the environment in which he or she lives. For some diseases the situation is quite clear, the person affected has inherited from one or both parents one or more genes which are associated with a particular problem. In other cases the inherited component is less important and only under certain conditions is the 'weakness' which has been inherited unmasked by some environmental upset. What of high blood pressure?

The lack of a clear dividing line between high and normal blood pressure makes it unlikely that a single gene determines the presence or absence of high blood pressure. Rather, the way blood pressure levels vary in the population suggests that it is under the control of a number of genes. Some people have low blood pressure, some high blood pressure, but the majority

High blood pressure is hereditary. If it runs in your family it is a good idea to make sure everyone has regular checks – including the children.

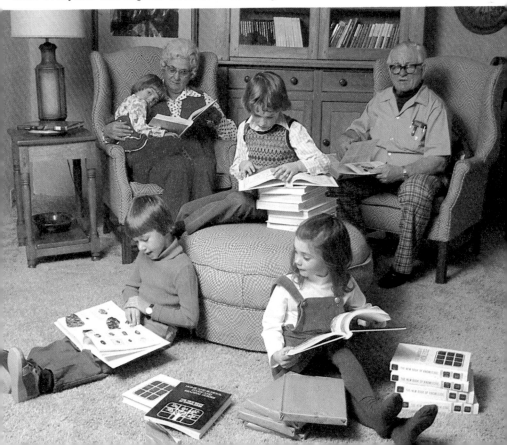

have pressure close to the average level.

Evidence concerning the role of inheritance in high blood pressure also comes from records of single families, studies of family histories and from comparisons of blood pressure in identical and non-identical twins. All these studies show that high blood pressure runs in families. The blood pressure of identical twins is more alike than that of non-identical twins. First-degree relatives of persons with high blood pressure have higher blood pressure than relatives of persons with normal blood pressure. Furthermore, children of parents with high blood pressure have higher pressure than the children of people with normal blood pressure.

New information on the genetic basis for high blood pressure has recently come from France. Researchers in Paris have produced evidence which suggests that people with high blood pressure have genetic defects of some enzymes or body chemicals involved in the handling of salt in the body. If this finding is confirmed, it may have considerable implications in future control, and possibly even prevention, of high blood pressure.

Because your doctor will be aware of the hereditary basis for high blood pressure he will almost certainly ask you if there is a history of high blood pressure in your family. When the family history of high blood pressure is particularly strong, it is generally worth making a special effort to have all members of your family checked. Even your children should have their blood pressure regularly measured. This is important, because the pattern is established in childhood and if preventive measures are to be taken, the earlier they are enforced the better.

Environmental factors

Salt Of the various environmental factors that have been implicated in high blood pressure none has been given as much attention as salt. Most Western populations eat three to ten times more salt than they need and if the causative role of salt in high blood pressure was definitely established, a public health campaign would be aimed at reducing salt consumption.

We shall look more closely at the part salt plays in our diet in chapter six, but it is worth mentioning here that in some countries with a very low salt consumption not only is high blood pressure very rare, but also blood pressure does not rise with age as seen in Western society.

Alcohol   The role of alcohol is difficult to assess, but studies from Birmingham in England indicate that blood pressure is raised in those who drink excessively. Alcoholics who remain 'dry' after withdrawal have a lower blood pressure than those who start drinking again. It seems, however, that those of us who are moderate or social drinkers are not at risk.

Obesity   Although obesity and high blood pressure are known to be related, it is not known if it is the obesity itself or some associated factor which is the cause of high blood pressure in those who are overweight.

Whatever the precise connection, it is clearly desirable for you to reduce if you are overweight; chapter six offers some advice about the best way to go about this.

Stress   Emotional stress at home or at work can cause a marked rise in blood pressure, but this is usually short-lived. There is no proof that repeated short periods of raised blood pressure lead to sustained high blood pressure, but obviously it is advisable for us to avoid prolonged periods of stress if possible. This, of course, is one aspect of our environment over which we generally do not have control, but later we will try to show you ways of relaxing and coping with stressful situations. (See chapter eight.)

Smoking   Smoking, like stress, causes temporary increases in blood pressure, but again there is no evidence that it produces sustained high blood pressure. However, smoking is one of the most serious risk factors for heart disease and stroke, and therefore people with high blood pressure who smoke are putting themselves at grave risk. That is why doctors strongly advise anyone with high blood pressure to give up smoking.

Tests you may be asked to have

Although we cannot discover a cause for the commonest form of high blood pressure, your doctor may often want some tests carried out. The purpose of these tests is to exclude the rare causes of 'secondary' high blood pressure, and to assess the general state of your heart, circulation and kidneys. These common and simple tests might include: urine tests, blood tests, the ECG (EKG in North America), the chest X-ray.

Urine tests   Examination of the urine for abnormalities is probably the oldest laboratory test used today. As the urine is formed by the kidney, defects in structure or function of the kidney are often revealed by the presence of abnormal constituents in the urine.

Most often the urine is tested using a strip of paper impregnated with chemicals which react to the urine by changing colour. Abnormalities in the amount of sugar, protein or blood and the presence of infection may be detected in this way. In addition the acidity of the urine can be estimated.

Further evaluation can be done if necessary by subjecting a sample of urine to a more rigorous laboratory examination. Sometimes it is necessary to obtain a sample when passing urine, and this is called a mid-stream or MSU test. The specimen is sent to the laboratory where it is examined under a microscope. It may also be cultured to ascertain the nature of any bacteria that may be present. If there are any abnormal findings further tests may be necessary – the most likely being the kidney X-ray.

Blood tests   Most people have had a blood sample taken at some time or other and you may remember the needle and syringe quite vividly. However, you will probably agree that the procedure is really quite trivial and not very uncomfortable. The blood is removed from the vein in the front of the elbow and may be examined for various substances.

As a general test of health the level of haemoglobin in the blood is measured. A low level indicates anaemia and requires further investigation.

Another test is also sometimes taken to assess whether the kidney is functioning properly. This means taking a measure of the level in the blood of chemicals called urea (also called blood urea nitrogen and abbreviated to BUN in North America) or creatinine. If the kidney is failing in its function these substances are not excreted in the urine as efficiently as they should be and they therefore accumulate in the blood.

The balance of potassium in the body may also be disturbed when kidney function is abnormal; the doctor may wish to check this as well as sugar, uric acid and fat levels in the blood.

The ECG   The electrocardiogram or ECG (EKG in North America) is a tracing of the electrical activity of the heart. In fact it is twelve tracings because various combinations of 'views' of

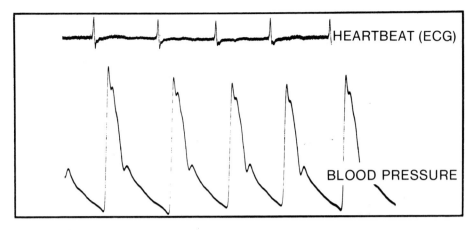

The upper trace, known as an electrocardiogram (ECG), is a record of electrical activity in the heart. The lower shows corresponding changes in blood pressure. The peaks represent systolic pressure; the troughs, diastolic.

the heart are obtained by changing the positions and combinations of the recording electrodes.

The ECG taken while you are at rest tells a good deal about how your blood pressure may have affected your heart. It may indicate that the elevated blood pressure has produced some strain on the heart and it will also tell your doctor something about the condition of your coronary arteries.

The chest X-ray The chest X-ray gives a fairly reliable indication of the size of the heart. In this respect it helps to confirm some of the findings seen on the ECG. In addition it may show signs that the heart is not pumping as well as it should.

High blood pressure with an identifiable cause

Now we will look at those rare cases (less than 5 per cent) in which it is possible to identify a definite cause for the raised blood pressure. Doctors call this condition 'secondary' high blood pressure.

Kidney conditions

Because of the central role of the kidney in controlling salt

35

elimination from the body it should come as no surprise that disorders of the kidney may lead to high blood pressure. Long-standing infection, narrowing of the arteries to the kidneys, failure of the kidney, and some other less common kidney conditions can result in high blood pressure, and X-ray tests will reveal if any of these problems are the cause of your high blood pressure.

An X-ray of the kidney is called an intravenous pyelogram, or IVP for short. A radio-opaque substance is used, that is, a substance through which X-rays will not pass, so that a white shadow appears on the X-ray. This substance, often incorrectly called a dye, is injected into an arm vein and it is rapidly taken up by the kidney and excreted. At different times in its passage through the kidney it outlines the tissues of the kidney and the system which collects the urine and conveys it to the bladder.

The contrast material throws into sharp relief any deformities of the collecting system as well as changes in size, position, shape or function of the kidney. Thus evidence of any damage due to infection or blockage will be revealed. Such abnormalities are present in most cases of 'secondary' high blood pressure. When detected further tests may be necessary, or occasionally an operation is required in order to put matters right.

If the IVP suggests that there is a decrease in the size of one of the kidneys or the renal artery, which carries blood to the kidneys, it may be necessary to take samples of blood coming from the kidney to measure the content of renin, a chemical involved in raising blood pressure (see page 16). This gives a good indication of whether the impression given by the X-ray is reflected in a true difference in renin output by the kidney on the affected side. If it turns out that this is so surgery may be required, but this is a highly specialized field.

Some doctors measure blood renin levels as a routine. To enable them to interpret the results more precisely they may also ask their patients to collect urine over a twenty-four-hour period. In this way renin levels can be related to the amount of salt in the urine.

Gland problems

Endocrine problems – that is problems to do with the glands – are rare. Overactivity of the adrenal gland (so-called because it is situated near the kidney) may result in a number of different abnormalities. An excess of the hormone aldosterone released from the gland causes salt and water retention and thereby increases blood pressure. Enlargement of the gland – a condition known as phaeochromocytoma – may result in excessive production of adrenaline (called epinephrine in North America) and noradrenaline (norepinephrine), and these hormones raise blood pressure by constricting blood vessels.

People suffering from any of these problems may look and feel flushed and have attacks of palpitation, headaches and sweating. The presence of any abnormality can be confirmed by measuring the amount of various chemicals in the urine over a twenty-four-hour period. Most forms of adrenal problems can be remedied by surgery, but special tests are generally carried out first.

Drugs

You must always tell your doctor if you are taking any drugs in addition to those prescribed by him, because these could themselves be causing high blood pressure. Or they may interfere with the action of the drugs prescribed by your doctor to lower your blood pressure. Drugs are an extremely important cause of high blood pressure; and by stopping them the problem is cured in the simplest way possible.

Even drugs bought over the counter without a prescription can cause high blood pressure. Cold remedies, for example, contain drugs capable of constricting blood vessels. This sometimes happens with nose drops (nasal decongestants), as the dose absorbed into the system through the nasal passages can be quite large. So do tell your doctor if you are using any medication he has not prescribed for you himself.

The pill Another commonly used drug which also raises blood pressure is, of course, the birth control pill. Most contain the hormones oestrogen and progesterone which may interfere with the renin system and cause salt retention with an increase in blood pressure. Most people who take the pill have an increase in blood pressure, but the increase is usually small and not sufficient to cause high blood pressure. But for some, perhaps those whose blood pressure is already 'high normal', the pill raises pressure sufficiently to cause high blood pressure.

While most cases are mild to moderate, even severe high blood pressure can occur. It is important, therefore, for anyone considering taking the pill to have her blood pressure checked first, and then to have it measured at regular intervals thereafter. For a fuller discussion of the pill and high blood pressure see chapter nine.

Oestrogens are also sometimes prescribed during the menopause. The dose used here is quite low and unlikely to cause high blood pressure, but it is a point to watch out for.

MAOI A group of drugs called mono-amine oxidase inhibitors (MAOI for short) are sometimes used to help treat depression. More commonly tricyclic antidepressant or newer mood-elevating drugs are given, but for some people who for one reason or another fail to respond to these the MAOI are prescribed. The MAOI have an effect on the activity of adrenaline.

A number of foods (wine, beer, cheese, relishes, pickles and yeast-and-vegetable extracts) contain tyramine. In the presence of MAOI tyramine releases excessive amounts of noradrenaline and adrenaline, and in addition the MAOI prevent the breakdown of these naturally occurring substances. Noradrenaline constricts the blood vessels and blood pressure increases. All patients who are prescribed MAOI are warned of this and given a list of foods and drinks known to contain tyramine. If you are taking MAOI and are in any doubt about a particular food you should consult your doctor.

Pregnancy
High blood pressure in pregnancy is generally considered to be secondary high blood pressure, but in fact we do not know why some pregnant women get high blood pressure and others do not. For a fuller discussion see chapter nine.

In conclusion let us say that there are many possible causes for high blood pressure. It seems likely that most cases are influenced by a combination of genetic and environmental factors. When doctors carry out tests these are aimed at ascertaining both the cause and the effects of high blood pressure in the individual concerned. Rarely (in less than 5 per cent) do they find secondary high blood pressure. Nevertheless, it is very important to find such cases because it may well be possible to cure them.

5 LIVING WITH HIGH BLOOD PRESSURE

In discussing the general measures which help to reduce blood pressure, we will naturally consider the important advisory role that the doctor plays, but in the end it is up to you. You will have to follow your doctor's recommendations and change your lifestyle accordingly. As we have said before, the control – or management, a term doctors sometimes use – of any long-term problem, such as high blood pressure, will only be successful if there is understanding and co-operation between you and your doctor. We believe, on the basis of our experience in dealing with people who have high blood pressure, that co-operation is much easier to achieve if the patient understands the importance of following advice. This is particularly true in the case of high blood pressure which, after all, does not usually cause symptoms.

It is understandable that an apparently healthy individual with high blood pressure might question the necessity for modifying some of the pleasurable aspects of modern life. Nonetheless, the recommendations which we have put forward in the next three chapters are of great importance, and in many ways play as vital a role as drugs. Indeed, many people with high blood pressure can bring their blood pressure down to normal by following these recommendations, and so avoid the need for drug treatment altogether.

It may sometimes seem to you as you read these chapters that some of our suggestions for modifying certain aspects of your lifestyle are unreasonable and unrealistic. Much will depend, of course, on your ability to readjust by, for example, stopping smoking, or reducing weight and taking exercise. Much also depends on your motivation and wish to improve your outlook for the future. It is here that we feel information and education about high blood pressure is of great importance. However, we realize that some people can follow medical advice to the letter and others are not so fortunate. This may not be merely a matter of will-power, but may be related to other factors such as occupation, hours of work, stresses and so on. We are also aware that old habits die hard and that every so often a person may revert to them. Nonetheless it is possible to achieve a great degree of improvement in people who care about their future, and we know that even if the perfect lifestyle is not achieved, a modest readjustment may yield considerable benefits in the years to come. Our overall aim is not necessarily total abstinence, but rather 'moderation in all things'.

Your lifestyle

In the last decade we have seen a great reawakening of interest in the healthy way of living. We say reawakening, because although our forefathers may not have been as aware as we are of the benefits of a healthy way of life, they did lead a healthier existence. They took more exercise since they did not have cars, and most of our predecessors smoked less.

The renewed interest in health is readily seen in the weight-conscious, slim youths of today, and in the jogging phenomenon which has swept Western society. Associated with this there is an increasing awareness of the proven dangers of smoking and the possibly harmful effects of excessive eating and drinking. In North America where the populus has taken very definite measures to improve its lifestyle, there has been a considerable reduction in deaths from heart attack.

However, we must preserve a balanced outlook and examine carefully the evidence for some of the measures which are advocated so strongly from time to time. Life, after all, is hard enough without placing unnecessary restrictions on some of its more enjoyable aspects. Sometimes, of course, we cannot produce definitive evidence that something is good or bad for us; for example, we do not know for sure whether reducing cholesterol in the diet is of benefit, although there is some evidence to suggest it might be. To prove that changing our diet will influence a disease such as hardening of the arteries (atherosclerosis), which develops from early life and perhaps does not manifest itself until old age, is often impossible.

Whenever there is scientific uncertainty over an important issue you will also invariably find two opposing schools of thought on the subject. Such is the state of affairs within the medical profession on the cholesterol question. One group believes that modifying our diet will be beneficial, and the other says not. So for the general reader who wants a positive recommendation, there is no straight answer. All that we can do in this situation is examine the facts, give a reasoned interpretation and make what seems to be the best decisions on the information available at the time.

There is, however, one aspect of modern living about which we need have no doubt about its harmful effects, and that is cigarette smoking.

Smoking – give it up

The havoc that smoking, especially cigarette smoking, has produced in modern society is truly alarming. Not only is smoking the major risk factor for disease of the heart and blood vessels, it is also the major cause of lung cancer (the death rate for smokers is eleven times higher than for non-smokers),

Cigarette smoking dramatically increases the risk of dying suddenly. For every 44 sudden deaths among non-smokers, there are 217 among heavy cigarette smokers.

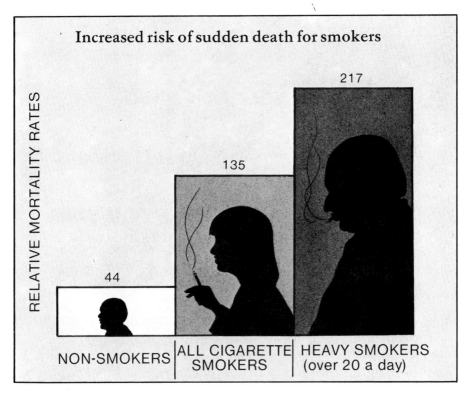

Increased risk of sudden death for smokers

RELATIVE MORTALITY RATES

217

135

44

NON-SMOKERS | ALL CIGARETTE SMOKERS | HEAVY SMOKERS (over 20 a day)

DISEASES CAUSED BY SMOKING
(From the report of the United States Surgeon General 1979)

Disease or condition	Comment
Death	Risk greatly increased for men and women. Male smokers have 70% greater risk than non-smokers. A thirty- to thirty-five-year-old, two pack-a-day smoker has a life expectancy eight to nine years shorter than a non-smoker of the same age. Pipe and cigar smokers have greater risk than non-smokers but less than cigarette smokers. Risk returns to normal after ten to fifteen years cessation of smoking.
Heart attack	Risk greatly increased. Main contributor to excess mortality. If you survive a heart attack and continue smoking the risk of recurrence is greatly increased. If you continue smoking and have a recurrence the risk of dying is increased fourfold.
Lung cancer	Risk greatly increased in men and women. Risk is proportional to the number of cigarettes smoked, duration of smoking, age of commencement, degree of inhalation, tar and nicotine content of cigarettes. Risk is less for pipe and cigar smokers but greater than for non-smokers.
Other lung diseases *Chronic bronchitis*	Smoking is the most important cause. Smoking greatly increases the risk of dying from bronchitis and emphysema.
Chronic sinusitis *Infections such as influenza* *Allergic disease*	Increased by smoking.
Other circulatory diseases *Peripheral vascular disease (of blood vessels near the skin)*	
Aneurysm of the aorta	Smoking increases the risk.
Blood pressure	Smoking does not cause high blood pressure but smoking and high blood pressure greatly increases risk of heart attack.

Other cancers
Larynx
Mouth
Oesophagus (gullet)   All have higher occurrence rate in smokers.
Bladder
Kidney
Pancreas

Peptic ulcer   Increased occurrence.
                               Death due to peptic ulcer is two times higher in smokers.
                               Smoking probably retards ulcer healing.

Effects on pregnancy
Birth weight   Mothers who smoke have lighter babies. The more the mother smokes the greater the reduction in birth weight.

Placental weight   Rate of placental to birth weight increases with increasing levels of maternal smoking, may mean reduced oxygen supply to foetus and affect survival.

Foetal growth   Retarded by smoking

Long-term growth   Smoking during pregnancy may affect physical growth, mental development, and behavioural characteristics of children up to age eleven.

Death around the time of birth   Risk is greater in mothers who smoke.

Preterm birth   Risk increased by smoking.

'Sudden infant death syndrome' (cot death)   Risk is higher in infants born to mothers who smoke.

Neonatal (newborn) death   Risk increased for a number of reasons in infants born to mothers who smoke.

Effects on work
Accidents   Smoking contributes to risk of accidents at work.

Miscellaneous   Smoking may act in combination with physical and chemical agents found in the work place to produce or increase a broad spectrum of adverse health effects.

Effects on others   Evidence is appearing that suggests that non-smokers may have increased risks for some illness through inhaling smoke involuntarily.
                               Children of parents who smoke are more likely to have bronchitis and pneumonia during the first year of life.

chronic bronchitis, emphysema, sinusitis and laryngitis; it has also been implicated in peptic ulceration and cancer of the bladder.

There is now some evidence that smokers may not only harm themselves, but also those unfortunate to be close enough to inhale the smoke from their cigarettes. Add to all this the fire hazard of smoking and one is left with a picture of human devastation which if brought about by fever epidemic would be viewed by the public with incredulity and alarm.

In spite of the awful statistics it has proved extraordinarily difficult to get people to give it up. Basically there are two reasons. First, there is the dependence, or if you prefer, the addiction, of the individual to tobacco; and secondly there is the financial dependence of most governments on the revenue generated by the sales of cigarettes and tobacco. So it is that many countries are faced with the unfortunate situation of paying enormous sums to treat the illnesses induced by cigarette smoking, and also providing finance for stop-smoking campaigns. Furthermore, there seems to be a reluctance to interfere too drastically with the price of cigarettes or the means used to advertise their sales.

Nonetheless, some encouraging signs have emerged that the sales of tobacco may finally be falling, but unfortunately there is as yet no strong evidence that health campaigns have influenced cigarette smoking in the young. The medical profession was, for obvious reasons, the first major group by and large to stop smoking and the beneficial effects of this have become apparent over the years.

A recent editorial in the *British Medical Journal* viewed the catastrophe of smoking as follows:

In the holocaust of the First World War almost a million British died. The scale of this tragic waste was a yardstick against which other disasters were measured until casualties from other wars and accounts of genocide in Nazi Germany and more recently South East Asia dulled reactions and made mass loss of life familiar. Yet all this time another avoidable holocaust has been going on ... between one and a half and three million Britons must have died prematurely from an avoidable cause; yet successive governments have shirked their responsibility and have done little to confront such a major threat to public health.

What are the consequences?

So much for the overall risk, what are the consequences for you? This makes an even more sorrowful litany:

Smoking twenty cigarettes a day doubles the risk of a coronary heart disease.

Cigarette smoking doubles the mortality from coronary heart disease.

Among men who smoke heavily, the risk of stroke is three times greater than in non-smokers.

The woman who smokes in her reproductive years may have an earlier menopause than normal, during pregnancy she has a greater tendency to spontaneous abortion, there may be increased infant mortality around the time of delivery, and her child may be of lower than average birth weight.

In Britain about a quarter of the 40,000 deaths in men and women under sixty-five who die each year from coronary heart disease are considered to be closely associated with cigarette smoking.

And so on and so on. The more we look at the statistics the more convinced we become that smoking *is* dangerous to health. Reports from the Surgeon General in the United States (see pages 42 and 43) and from the Royal College of Physicians in London all support unequivocally the conclusion that cigarette smoking shortens life expectancy and that it is a major cause of illness and premature death in Western society.

What does smoking do to the circulation?

Smoking may cause increased hardening of the arteries (atherosclerosis); it may have a direct effect on the heart muscle, or induce clotting changes in the blood; or it may increase circulating adrenaline and cause disturbances of heart rhythm, very occasionally with serious consequences.

Although smoking increases blood pressure temporarily, it has not been shown to be a cause of high blood pressure. However, the most serious form of high blood pressure, known as accelerated or malignant hypertension, is commoner in smokers than non-smokers, and is more likely to follow a lethal course in the former group. And it is known that high blood pressure and smoking are the two most dangerous risk factors operating on the heart and blood vessels, and that they increase the likelihood of stroke and heart attack many times. It is therefore at least as important for you to stop smoking as it is to have effective treatment for your raised blood pressure.

What happens if you give up smoking?

If you want to stop smoking it is important to realize at the outset that first, tobacco is an addictive drug, which means you have probably become dependent on it; and so when you stop you will have withdrawal symptoms. Second, you must have a very genuine desire to stop the habit, and this means being in a sufficiently determined frame of mind.

Perhaps it should also be said that there do not appear to be any thoroughly proven successful aids to giving up cigarettes. Many efforts have been made to develop something to make the break easier: there have been substitute cigarettes, efforts have been made at hypnosis, and lately there has been nicotine gum. All these measures have had varying success, but it would seem that the most important factor is the determination of the individual, and an understanding of the problems that lie ahead.

When advised to give up cigarettes completely a person has three options: he can walk from the doctor's office, throw away the cigarettes that remain in his packet and vow never to smoke again; he can think about his doctor's advice and perhaps postpone the decision until he feels circumstances are more conducive to success (he might be under a lot of stress at work, or he might have a vacation coming up which would be a better time for him to stop); or he might decide to reduce gradually, possibly with the help of some of the aids mentioned above, in the hope of ultimately giving up cigarettes, or at least reducing his consumption considerably. Whichever course is decided upon, and any one might be successful depending on the individual, belief in the benefit of giving up smoking is essential.

We feel that perhaps the best thing is to strike while the iron is hot and stop as soon as the advice is given, but this may not be the best course if you have stresses at home or work or are likely, for example, to be travelling a lot or entertaining in the near future. Any of these factors may make success more difficult. You should try to choose a time when family and home circumstances are tranquil, and when the social circumstances seem appropriate. It might not be a good idea to try to give up smoking at Christmas, whereas the New Year might be more suitable. It is probably as well to avoid heavy drinking of alcohol when trying to stop smoking because alcohol considerably reduces one's determination.

Let us assume that you succeed. In all likelihood you will have done more to improve your future outlook than any medicine can ever do. We know that high blood pressure is a major risk factor for stroke and heart disease, and we also know that cigarette smoking is another major risk factor for these diseases. When both these factors are present the risk is not merely doubled, it is probably trebled or even quadrupled, but if we can remove both risk factors we can assume that the benefit is correspondingly great.

Do's and don'ts

For those who cannot stop completely the following guidelines may be helpful (based on the Joint Working Party of the Royal College of Physicians of London and the British Cardiac Society):

Smoke less than five cigarettes daily.

Smoke filter cigarettes of low tar and nicotine content using the Government Tar and Nicotine Tables.

Try not to inhale.

Do not smoke in front of your children (the majority of teenagers who start smoking become established adult smokers).

Change from cigarettes to a pipe or cigars, keeping your consumption as low as possible.

A few words of caution here: it is generally accepted that the risk from smoking a pipe or cigars is less than for cigarette smoking, and it is certainly true that the mortality rate is lower. However, the technique of the cigarette smoker is often quite different from that of the person who has always smoked cigars or a pipe. The cigarette smoker inhales more and when he changes over to a pipe or cigars he manages to get more nicotine into his blood than the pipe or cigar smoker. So it may be that he will not improve his situation all that much by changing, especially if he continues to use large amounts of tobacco.

When smoking is stopped completely there is a fall in the mortality for coronary disease in the first year, but it may take ten years or more for the death rate to slow down to that of people who have always been non-smokers. Therefore the sooner you stop the better.

6 TAKE CARE OF YOUR DIET

Many items in our diet have been implicated in blood circulation problems, but only a few have been proved to have a significant role. Of the dietary factors we shall look at here the most important are the calorie, salt, cholesterol and saturated fat content of foodstuffs.

By calories we mean the energy content of food. Ideally we should consume just enough calories for our daily needs. Those of us who lead very energetic lives or do a great deal of physical exercise require considerably more calories than those whose occupation is sedentary – office workers, for example. If our calorie intake is excessive, the excess calories are converted into fat and over the years this leads to obesity.

Obesity – why it matters

In the past obesity has been regarded as something of a social inevitability, whereas in reality it is a disease, and a very serious one. Obesity contributes to the hardening of the arteries – atherosclerosis – that underlies stroke and coronary heart disease; it contributes to high blood pressure; it is often the cause of diabetes in later life; it makes us less agile and more accident-prone; it contributes to bronchitis; and, of course, in time the body scaffolding – the skeleton – cannot cope with the extra strain, and arthritis, backache and varicose veins develop. Also, fat people have a shorter life expectancy.

The problem is widespread; it has been estimated that about one-third of the adult population in Britain, North America and Australia are above the maximum desirable weight.

The effects of obesity on the circulatory system can be explained in a fairly simple way. The heart has to pump blood to each tiny fragment of tissue in the body sixty to seventy times a minute, every minute of the day, every day of the year, throughout our lives. One does not need to be a brilliant mathematician to visualize the increased workload for the heart in having to pump blood around an extra 10 or 20lb of useless fatty tissue sixty to seventy times per minute throughout our lives. And if we were to assess the heart in purely mechanical terms, as we would a motor car for instance, we might not be too far out in assuming that it has a life of so many pumping minutes, in much the same way as the motor car has a life of so many driving miles. If we choose to use up the heart's working

There is a clear relationship between obesity and increasing death rates. The average death rate for the population is 100.

Obesity as a risk factor

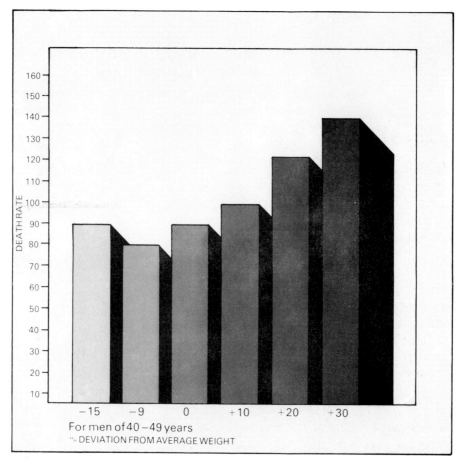

For men of 40 – 49 years

% DEVIATION FROM AVERAGE WEIGHT

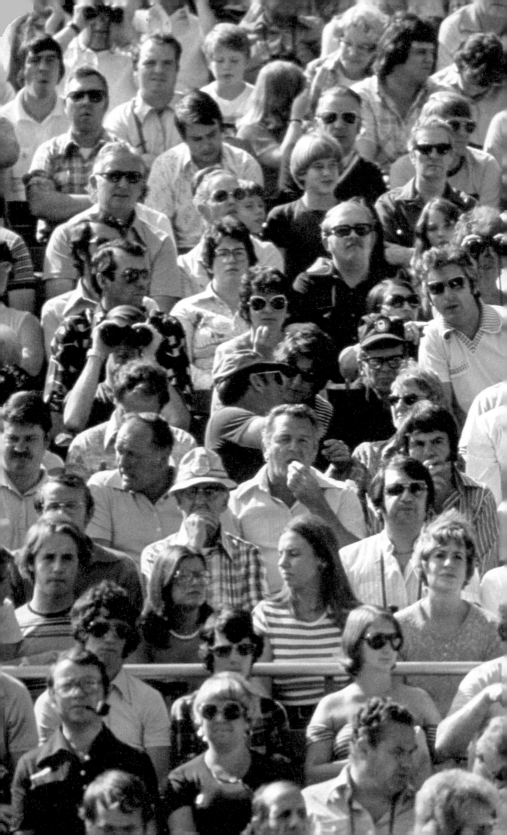

life in providing blood to useless fatty tissue, we must expect to shorten its total life.

Life insurance companies have known for many decades that overweight people have a shorter life expectancy and are not profitable to insure. John S. Garrow of the Clinical Research Centre at Northwick Park Hospital in England, when reviewing the subject recently observed: 'Without any doubt, then, overweight people tend to die sooner than their lean contemporaries; ... the life insurance experience suggests that the association between overweight and excess mortality is reversible if weight is lost and is preventable by preventing obesity.' So it obviously makes good sense to lose weight if you are above the maximum for your height and frame (see overleaf).

In the Framingham Study (see page 18) – one of the best population surveys on the topic – it was shown that three times more people with normal blood pressure who were overweight developed higher blood pressure than expected. In the same study it was also demonstrated that a weight loss of 15 per cent or more in men was associated with an average 10 per cent decrease in systolic blood pressure. Other studies have given similar results and have shown that people with high blood pressure who reduce weight need fewer drugs to control their blood pressure.

How to find your ideal weight

Over the years tables of ideal weights have been produced, based mostly on figures from insurance companies. These tables are divided into large, medium and small frame sizes and there are separate figures for men and women (see overleaf).

Dr John Garrow maintains that weight would be better and more simply determined by using the formula $\frac{W}{H^2}$ where W is the person's weight in kilograms and H the height in metres. He has calculated the normal ranges for $\frac{W}{H^2}$ to be: Men: 20–25; Women: 19–24.

If you are a man weighing 82 kg (180 lb) and are 1.83 m (6 ft) tall, you can determine if you are overweight by using the equation thus: square your height (1.83×1.83) which gives you 3.34, then divide this figure into your weight in kilograms $(82 \div 3.34)$ which gives you 24.5. This is within the desired range. If,

OPPOSITE: The chances are that one adult in three in this photograph is overweight.

Weight table for men of 25 years and over (in indoor clothing)

Height ft in	(cm)	Small frame lb	kg	Medium frame lb	kg	Large frame lb	kg
5 1	(155)	112–120	(51–54)	118–129	(54–59)	126–141	(57–64)
5 2	(157)	115–123	(52–56)	121–133	(55–60)	129–144	(59–65)
5 3	(160)	118–126	(54–57)	124–136	(56–62)	132–148	(60–67)
5 4	(163)	121–129	(55–58)	127–139	(58–63)	135–152	(61–69)
5 5	(165)	124–133	(56–60)	130–143	(59–65)	138–156	(63–71)
5 6	(168)	128–137	(58–62)	134–147	(61–67)	142–161	(64–73)
5 7	(170)	132–141	(60–64)	138–152	(63–69)	147–166	(67–75)
5 8	(173)	136–145	(62–66)	142–156	(64–71)	151–170	(68–77)
5 9	(175)	140–150	(63–68)	146–160	(66–73)	155–174	(70–79)
5 10	(178)	144–154	(65–70)	150–165	(68–75)	159–179	(72–81)
5 11	(180)	148–158	(67–72)	154–170	(70–77)	164–184	(74–83)
6 0	(183)	152–162	(69–74)	158–175	(72–80)	168–189	(76–86)
6 1	(185)	156–167	(71–76)	162–180	(74–82)	173–194	(78–88)
6 2	(188)	160–171	(73–78)	167–185	(76–84)	178–199	(81–90)
6 3	(190)	164–175	(74–80)	172–190	(78–86)	182–204	(83–92)

Weight table for women aged 25 and over (in indoor clothing)

(For women aged between 18 and 25 subtract 1 lb ($\frac{1}{2}$ kg) for each year under 25)

Height ft in	(cm)	Small frame lb	kg	Medium frame lb	kg	Large frame lb	kg
4 8	(142)	92–98	(42–44)	96–107	(44–49)	104–119	(47–54)
4 9	(145)	94–101	(43–46)	98–110	(45–50)	106–122	(48–55)
4 10	(147)	96–104	(44–47)	101–113	(46–51)	109–125	(49–57)
4 11	(150)	99–107	(45–48)	104–116	(47–53)	112–128	(51–58)
5 0	(152)	102–110	(46–50)	107–119	(48–54)	115–131	(52–59)
5 1	(155)	105–113	(48–51)	110–122	(50–55)	118–134	(53–60)
5 2	(157)	108–116	(49–53)	113–126	(51–57)	121–138	(55–63)
5 3	(160)	111–119	(50–54)	116–130	(53–59)	125–142	(57–64)
5 4	(163)	114–123	(52–56)	120–135	(54–61)	129–146	(58–66)
5 5	(165)	118–127	(53–58)	124–139	(56–63)	133–150	(60–68)
5 6	(168)	122–131	(55–59)	128–143	(58–65)	137–154	(62–70)
5 7	(170)	126–135	(57–61)	132–147	(60–67)	141–158	(64–72)
5 8	(173)	130–140	(59–63)	136–151	(62–69)	145–163	(66–74)
5 9	(175)	134–144	(61–65)	140–155	(63–70)	149–168	(68–76)
5 10	(178)	138–148	(63–67)	144–159	(65–72)	153–173	(69–78)

however, your weight was 96 kg (210 lb) the result would be 28 which is outside the desired range.

This method has the virtue of simplicity, and although it is not yet generally accepted it may be more accurate and could become popular. Most of us, of course, know when we are overweight by our appearance or by comparing our present weight with our weight in our teens. Some of us, however, have had to fight the calorie battle ever since childhood.

There are other methods of assessing obesity, such as measuring skinfold thickness with a special instrument. A simpler test is to lean forward slightly and pinch up a fold of skin over your stomach, just below the rib cage. If this is an inch (2.5 cm) or more you should lose some weight.

How to lose weight

Putting on weight is an insidious process that goes on gradually over many years. We may be consuming too many calories for our particular exertional needs during our twenties and perhaps our thirties, and quite suddenly in our mid-thirties or early forties we realize we have a weight problem, sometimes a serious one. Then there begins the struggle with diet in an effort to get back to our normal weight.

By this time, however, it is not just a question of reducing our calorie consumption, it is a matter of changing a long-established lifestyle in relation to eating. As with a bank overdraft, it is easy to borrow and so difficult to pay back. With today's slim-conscious youth – perhaps more for reasons of fashion than of health – it is possible that the problem of overeating and middle-aged obesity will not be as great in future generations.

People in Western society tend to overeat by consuming not only too many calories at each meal, but also by eating too many meals each day. Many of us have two large meals a day in addition to a large breakfast, whereas one main meal with a light snack either at breakfast, lunch or supper (depending on when you like your main meal) is quite sufficient. Some dietitians say that three small meals a day is best; but however many you take remember that calorie intake is not confined to food alone, and that there is a very high calorie content in most alcoholic beverages, as well as in many soft drinks. So we not only have to watch what we eat, but also what we drink.

Avoid slimming drugs

It is not easy to lose weight, but the success rates do seem to be better than for giving up cigarettes. Again, there must be determination and a genuine desire to reduce weight. As with cigarette smoking, many attempts have been made to provide the would-be slimmer with various aids to help weight reduction, but a number of these have been harmful rather than helpful. However, the many self-help groups and slimming clubs that exist are of great benefit in reinforcing determination and indeed, for some, participation in such groups is the only way to success. But we have no hesitation in condemning outright the use of anoretic (appetite-suppressing) drugs, hormonal preparations and diuretics (water-losing pills) as aids for losing weight. Their effects, if any, are very brief and there are significant risks if you use them.

The sensible way to lose weight is gradually. Chose a diet low in calories that suits your taste.

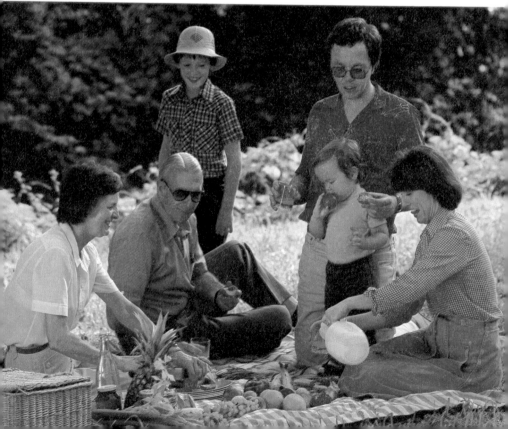

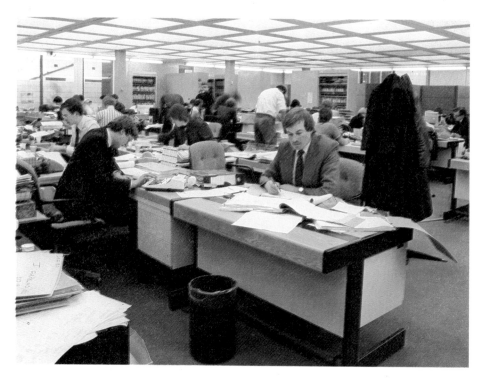

To maintain a healthy body weight a sedentary office worker needs only about half the daily calorie intake of someone whose job involves strenuous exercise.

The diet

There has been a tendency to promote fixed diets, with a choice of menu for breakfast, lunch and dinner, but we do not advocate this approach. We believe it is better for each person to choose a diet which suits his or her particular likes and dislikes, according to means, and in keeping with the dictates of their culture and religion. We have therefore included a table (pages 56 to 59) giving the calorie content of different foods and drinks from which you can devise your own dietary regimen. Once again we would draw attention to the high calorie content of alcohol, and emphasize that everything you eat, including beverages and snacks must be calculated and included in the total daily calorie count.

Watch the calories

For most people leading a sedentary life, a daily intake of 1,200 calories will suffice and to lose weight you would have to keep to

Guide to calorie values for the UK, Ireland and Australia

Dairy products   Calories

Butter 1 oz (30 g)	220
Cheese, Cheddar 1 oz (30 g)	120
cream 1 oz (30 g)	100
low fat, cottage 1 oz (30 g)	30
thickened 1 oz (30 g)	95
reduced 1 oz (30 g)	80
Egg fried or scrambled 2 oz (60 g)	135
poached or boiled 2 oz (60 g)	93
Low-fat spread 1 oz (30 g)	105
Margarine 1 oz (30 g)	220
Milk, dried, skimmed 1 oz (30 g)	95
fresh, skimmed ½ pt (300 ml)	100
fresh, whole ½ pt (300 ml)	190
Yogurt flavoured 1 oz (30 g)	30
natural 1 oz (30 g)	20
natural, non-fat 1 oz (30 g)	15

Meat and poultry

Bacon, grilled 4 oz (125 g)	700
gammon rashers 4 oz (125 g)	520
Beef corned 4 oz)125 g)	280
roast, lean 4 oz (125 g)	255
steak, grilled 4 oz (125 g)	330
Chicken, av roast 4 oz (125 g)	250
boiled 4 oz (125 g)	220
Duck, roast 4 oz (125 g)	350
Frankfurters 4 oz (125 g)	290
Goose, roast 4 oz (125 g)	370
Ham, lean, boiled 4 oz (125 g)	250
Hamburger 1 medium	125
Kidneys, grilled 4 oz (125 g)	130
Lamb, chop, lean, grilled 4 oz (125 g)	310
chop, fried 4 oz (125 g)	340
Lamb, av roast 4 oz (125 g)	450
lean, dry roast 4 oz (125 g)	350
Liver, grilled 4 oz (125 g)	180
Pork chop, lean, grilled 4 oz (125 g)	400
Sausages, beef, thick, grilled 4 oz (125 g)	280
pork, thick, grilled 4 oz (125 g)	330
Sausage roll 4 oz (125 g)	300
Tongue 4 oz (125 g)	115
Tripe 4 oz (125 g)	125
Turkey, av roast 4 oz (125 g)	340
dry roast 4 oz (125 g)	240
Veal 4 oz (125 g)	220

Fish

Bream 4 oz (125 g)	160
Cod, fillets, baked 4 oz (125 g)	95
fillets, grilled 4 oz (125 g)	95
Flounder 4 oz (125 g)	120
Haddock, smoked, poached 4 oz (125 g)	128
Halibut 4 oz (125 g)	160
Herring, fried 4 oz (125 g)	270
grilled 4 oz (125 g)	190
tinned, plain 4 oz (125 g)	250
tinned, in tomato sauce 4 oz (125 g)	220
Kipper grilled 4 oz (125 g)	200
Lobster 4 oz (125 g)	115
Mackerel, grilled 4 oz (125 g)	200
Oysters ½ doz	40
Pilchard, tinned 4 oz (125 g)	180
Plaice, steamed 4 oz (125 g)	100
Prawns 4 oz (125 g)	100
Salmon, fresh 4 oz (125 g)	160
tinned 4 oz (125 g)	160
Sardines, tinned 4 oz (125 g)	320
Scallops 4 oz (125 g)	100
Shrimps, fresh 4 oz (125 g)	110
Snapper 4 oz (125 g)	120
Sole, steamed 4 oz (125 g)	90
Trout 4 oz (125 g)	160
Tuna, tinned, in oil, drained 4 oz (125 g)	225
tinned, in brine, drained 4 oz (125 g)	150
Whiting, boiled 4 oz (125 g)	120

Vegetables

Asparagus 4 oz (125 g)	20
Aubergines 4 oz (125 g)	30
Avocado pear, half medium	185
Beans, baked, tinned 4 oz (125 g)	130
broad 4 oz (125 g)	50
French, boiled 4 oz (125 g)	40
runner, boiled 4 oz (125 g)	40
Beetroot, boiled 4 oz (125 g)	40
Broccoli, boiled 4 oz (125 g)	30
Brussel sprouts, boiled 4 oz (125 g)	50
Cabbage, boiled 4 oz (125 g)	30
Capsicum 4 oz (125 g)	45
Carrots, boiled 4 oz (125 g)	40
Cauliflower, boiled 4 oz (125 g)	30
Celery, raw 4 oz (125 g)	20
Cucumber 4 oz (125 g)	20
Leeks 4 oz (125 g)	50
Lettuce 4 oz (125 g)	20
Mushrooms, grilled 4 oz (125 g)	35
Onions, boiled 4 oz (125 g)	40
Parsley 4 oz (125 g)	Nil
Parsnips, boiled 4 oz (125 g)	80
Peas, fresh, boiled 4 oz (125 g)	90
tinned, drained 4 oz (125 g)	100
Potatoes, boiled 4 oz (125 g)	90
chipped, fried 4 oz (125 g)	270
crisps 4 oz (125 g)	680
Radish 4 oz (125 g)	20
Spinach, boiled 4 oz (125 g)	30
Sweetcorn 4 oz (125 g)	105
Tomatoes, fresh 4oz (125 g)	20
Turnips, boiled 4 oz (125 g)	35
Watercress 4 oz (125 g)	25

	Calories
Fruit	
Apple, baked *1 large*	100
fresh *1 medium (150 g)*	85
Apricot, dried *4 oz (125 g)*	300
Banana *1 medium (150 g)*	125
Cantaloupe melon *4 oz (125 g)*	35
Cherries, fresh *4 oz (125 g)*	90
Currants, dried *4 oz (125 g)*	320
Dates, pitted *4 oz (125 g)*	350
Figs, dried *4 oz (125 g)*	320
fresh *4 oz (125 g)*	100
Grapefruit, canned *4 oz (125 g)*	90
fresh *4 oz (125 g)*	50
Grapes *4 oz (125 g)*	80
Orange, fresh *4 oz (125 g)*	60
Peach, fresh *4 oz (125 g)*	50
tinned, sweetened *4 oz (125 g)*	85
Pineapple, fresh *4 oz (125 g)*	65
Plums, fresh *4 oz (125 g)*	75
Prunes, stewed *4 oz (125 g)*	220
Raisins, dried *4 oz (125 g)*	320
Raspberries, fresh *4 oz (125 g)*	70
Strawberries, fresh *4 oz (125 g)*	45
Sultanas, dried *4 oz (125 g)*	320
Watermelon *4 oz (125 g)*	30

	Calories
Puddings	
Blancmange *4 oz (125 g)*	140
Custard *4 oz (125 g)*	130
Ice Cream *4 oz (125 g)*	220
Jelly *4 oz (125 g)*	90
Rice pudding *4 oz (125 g)*	170
Sago pudding *4 oz (125 g)*	185
Semolina pudding *4 oz (125 g)*	400
Trifle *4 oz (125 g)*	180

	Calories
Biscuits, breads, cakes and cereals	
Biscuits, chocolate *2 oz (60 g)*	260
crispbread *2 oz (60 g)*	215
sweet *2 oz (60 g)*	260
Bread, brown *1 oz (30 g)*	70
white *1 oz (30 g)*	70
Cake, cheese *4 oz (125 g)*	350
fruit *2 oz (60 g)*	215
sponge *2 oz (60 g)*	185
Cereals, Allbran *1 oz (30 g)*	90
cornflakes *1 oz (30 g)*	105
oatmeal *1 oz (30 g)*	115
porridge *5 oz (155 g)*	85

	Calories
Doughnuts *2 oz (60 g)*	225
Dumplings *2 oz (60 g)*	120
Flour, cornflour *1 oz (30 g)*	100
white *1 oz (30 g)*	100
wholemeal *1 oz (30 g)*	100
Macaroni, boiled *2 oz (60 g)*	65
Pastries *2 oz (60 g)*	250
Rice, boiled *2 oz (60 g)*	70
Scones *2 oz (60 g)*	210
Spaghetti, boiled *2 oz (60 g)*	65
Yorkshire pudding *2 oz (60 g)*	75

	Calories
Miscellaneous	
Chocolate *1 oz (30 g)*	160
Gravy, thick *1 teaspoon*	35
Honey, jam and syrup *1 tablespoon*	75
Mayonnaise *1 tablespoon*	80
Peanuts, shelled *1 oz (30 g)*	170
Soup, clear *1 bowl (250 ml)*	35
thick *1 bowl (250 ml)*	100
Sugar $\frac{1}{2}$ *oz (15 g)*	55

	Calories
Drinks	
1. Alcohol	
Beer $\frac{1}{2}$ *pt 10 fl oz (300 ml)*	120
Champagne *10 fl oz (300 ml)*	245
Cider $\frac{1}{2}$ *pt 10 fl oz (300 ml)*	120
Gin, whisky, brandy, rum *1 fl oz (30 ml)*	65
Liqueurs *1 fl oz (30 ml)*	110
Sherry, sweet *1 fl oz (30 ml)*	45
dry *1 fl oz (30 ml)*	35
Stout *10 fl oz (300 ml)*	120
Wine, red *10 fl oz (300 ml)*	250
white, dry *10 fl oz (300 ml)*	230

	Calories
2. Non-alcoholic drinks	
Cocoa, with milk *1 cup (250 ml)*	185
Coffee, black *1 cup (250 ml)*	Negligible
milk and sugar (1 tspn) *1 cup (250 ml)*	40
Orange juice, fresh *1 glass (150 ml)*	65
Soft drinks *1 glass (150 ml)*	80
Tea, milk and sugar (1 tspn) *1 cup (250 ml)*	40
milk, no sugar *1 cup (250 ml)*	20
Tomato juice *1 glass (150 ml)*	30

Guide to calorie values for North America

1 cup equals 8 fluid ounces, 3 teaspoons (tsp) equal 1 tablespoon (tbs), 4 tablespoons (tbs) equal $\frac{1}{4}$ cup.

Dairy products

	Calories
Butter *1 tbs*	95
Cheese American Cheddar *1 cube*	
¹/₈ in sq	
or *3 tbs grated*	110
cottage *5 tbs*	100
cream *2 tbs*	100
Cream light *2 tbs*	65
heavy *2 tbs*	120
Custard boiled or baked $\frac{1}{2}$ *cup*	130
Egg *1 medium size*	75
Margarine *1 tbs*	100
Milk buttermilk (fat free) *1 cup*	85
condensed *1$\frac{1}{2}$ tbs*	100
evaporated $\frac{1}{2}$ *cup (1 cup diluted)*	160
whole milk, fresh *1 cup*	170
yoghurt, plain *1 cup*	120–160

Meat and poultry

	Calories
Bacon *2–3 long slices, cooked*	100
Bacon fat *1 tbs*	100
Beef corned *1 slice 4 x 1$\frac{1}{2}$ x 1 in*	100
dried *2 oz*	100
hamburger *1 patty (3 oz)*	300
round, lean *1 med slice (2 oz)*	125
sirloin, lean *1 av slice (3 oz)*	250
tongue *2 oz*	125
Chicken broiled $\frac{1}{2}$ *med broiler*	270
roast *1 slice 4 x 2$\frac{1}{2}$ x $\frac{1}{4}$ in*	100
Frankfurter *1 sausage*	125
Ham, lean *1 slice 4$\frac{1}{4}$ x 4 x $\frac{1}{2}$ in*	265
Lamb, roast *1 slice 3$\frac{1}{2}$ x 4$\frac{1}{2}$ x ¹/₈ in*	100
Lard *1 tbs*	100
Liver *1 slice 3 x 3 x $\frac{1}{2}$ in*	100
Liverwurst *2 oz*	130
Pork chop, lean *1 med*	200
Turkey, lean *1 slice 4 x 2$\frac{1}{2}$ x $\frac{1}{4}$ in*	100
Veal, roast *1 slice 3 x 3$\frac{3}{4}$ x $\frac{1}{2}$ in*	120

Fish

	Calories
Clams, *6 round*	100
Cod-steak, *1 piece 3$\frac{1}{2}$ x 2 x 1 in*	100
Halibut, *1 piece 3 x 1³/₈ x 1 in*	100
Oysters, *5 med*	100
Salmon, canned $\frac{1}{2}$ *cup*	100
Sardines, drained *5 fish 3 in long*	100
Tuna fish, canned $\frac{1}{4}$ *cup drained*	100

Vegetables

	Calories
Asparagus, fresh or canned *5 stalks 5 in long*	15
Avocado, $\frac{1}{2}$ *pear*	185
Beans, dried $\frac{1}{2}$ *cup, cooked*	135
lima, fresh or canned $\frac{1}{2}$ *cup*	100
Beet greens $\frac{1}{2}$ *cup cooked*	30
Beets *2 beets 2 in diam*	50
Broccoli *3 stalks 5$\frac{1}{2}$ in long*	100
Brussel sprouts *6 – 1$\frac{1}{2}$ in in diam*	50

	Calories
Cabbage, cooked $\frac{1}{2}$ *cup*	40
raw *1 cup*	25
Carrots, 1 carrot *4 in long*	25
Cauliflower $\frac{3}{4}$ *of a head 4$\frac{1}{4}$ in in diam*	25
Celery *2 stalks*	15
Chinese cabbage *1 cup raw*	20
Cooking fats, vegetable *1 tbs*	100
Cucumber $\frac{1}{2}$ *med*	10
Endive *average serving*	10
Kale $\frac{1}{2}$ *cup, cooked*	50
Lettuce *2 lge leaves*	5
Mushrooms *10 lge*	10
Onions *3–4 medium*	100
Parsnips *1 parsnip 7 in long*	100
Peas, canned $\frac{1}{2}$ *cup*	65
fresh shelled $\frac{3}{4}$ *cup*	100
Pepper, green *1 medium*	20
Potato chips *8–10 lge*	100
Potato salad with mayonnaise $\frac{1}{2}$ *cup*	200
Potatoes, mashed $\frac{1}{2}$ *cup*	100
sweet $\frac{1}{2}$ *medium*	100
white *1 medium*	100
Radishes *5*	10
Sauerkraut $\frac{1}{2}$ *cup*	15
Spinach $\frac{1}{2}$ *cup, cooked*	20
Squash, summer $\frac{1}{2}$ *cup, cooked*	20
winter $\frac{1}{2}$ *cup cooked*	50
Tomatoes, canned $\frac{1}{2}$ *cup*	25
fresh *1 medium*	30
Turnip *1 – 1$\frac{3}{4}$ in in diam*	25
Turnip greens $\frac{1}{2}$ *cup cooked*	30

Fruits

	Calories
Apples, baked *1 lge and 2 tbs sugar*	200
fresh *1 lge*	100
Apple sauce, sweetened $\frac{1}{2}$ *cup*	100
Apricots, canned in syrup *3 lge halves and 2 tbs juice*	100
dried *10 sm halves*	100
Banana *1 med, 6 in*	90
Blackberries, fresh *1 cup*	100
Cantaloupe $\frac{1}{2}$ *of a 5$\frac{1}{2}$ in melon*	50
Cherries, sweet *15 lge*	75
Cranberry sauce $\frac{1}{4}$ *cup*	100
Dates *4*	100
Figs, dried *3 small*	100
Grapefruit $\frac{1}{2}$ *medium*	50
Grapes, American or Tokay *1 bunch – 22 av*	75
seedless *1 bunch – 30 av*	75
Olives, green *4 med or 3 extra large*	15
Orange *1 med*	80
Peaches, canned in syrup *2 lge halves and 3 tbs juice*	100
fresh *1 med*	50
Pears, canned in syrup *3 halves and 3 tbs juice*	100
fresh *1 med*	50
Pineapple, fresh *1 slice $\frac{3}{4}$ in thick*	50

Calories

Plums, canned 2 *med and 1 tbs juice* 75
    fresh *2 med* 50
Prunes, dried *4 med* 100
Pumpkin ½ *cup* 50
Raisins ¼ *cup* 90
Raspberries, fresh *1 cup* 90
Rhubarb, stewed and sweetened ½
    cup 100
Strawberries, fresh *1 cup* 90
Tangerines *1 med* 60
Watermelon *1 round slice 6 in in*
    diam, 1½ in thick 190

Cakes, cookies, breads and cereals

Biscuit, *2 in in diam* 100
Breads, Boston brown *1 slice 3 in in*
    diam ¾ in thick 90
    corn (1-egg) *2 in square* 120
    cracked wheat *1 slice av* 80
    dark rye *1 slice ½ in thick* 70
    light rye *1 slice ½ in thick* 75
    white enriched *1 slice thin* 55
    wholewheat 100% *1 slice*
    av 75
Cake, chocolate or vanilla with no
    icing *1 piece 2 x 2 x 2 in* 200
    chocolate or vanilla with
    icing *1 piece 2 x 1½ x 2 in* 200
Corn ½ *cup* 70
Corn syrup *1 tbs* 75
Corn flakes *1 cup* 80
Corn meal *1 tbs uncooked* 35
Cornstarch pudding ½ *cup* 200
Crackers, graham *1 square* 35
    round snack-type *1*
    cracker 2 in in diam 15
    rye wafers *1 wafer* 25
    saltines *1 cracker 2 in sq* 15
Flour, white or whole grain *1 tbs*
    unsifted 35
Gingerbread, hot water *2 x 2 x 2 in* 200
Hominy grits ¾ *cup cooked* 100
Macaroni ¾ *cup cooked* 100
Muffins, bran *1 med* 90
    1-egg *1 med* 130
Noodles ¾ *cup cooked* 75
Oatmeal ¾ *cup cooked* 110
Pies, apple *3 in sector* 200
    lemon meringue *3 in sector* 300
    mincemeat *3 in sector* 300
    pumpkin *3 in sector* 250
Popcorn, plain *1½ cups popped* 100
Rice ¾ *cup cooked* 100
Waffles, *1 waffle 6 in in diam* 250
Wheat, flakes ¾ *cup* 100
    germ *1 tbs* 25
    shredded *1 biscuit* 100

Miscellaneous

Almonds *12–15* 100
Cashew nuts *4–5* 100

Calories

Chocolate, milk sweetened *1 oz* 140
    fudge *1 piece 1 in sq x ¾*
    in thick 100
    malted milk *fountain*
    size 460
Gelatin, fruit flavored, dry *3 oz pkg* 330
Hickory nuts *12–15* 100
Honey *1 tbs* 100
Ice cream ½ *cup* 200
Ice cream soda *fountain size* 325
Jellies and jams *1 rounded tbs* 100
Maple syrup *1 tbs* 70
Molasses *1 tbs* 70
Oil – corn, cottonseed, olive,
    peanut, sunflower *1 tbs* 100
Peanut butter *1 tbs* 100
Peanuts, shelled *10* 50
Pecans *6* 100
Pickles, cucumber sour and dill *10*
    slices *2 in in diam* 10
    sweet *1 small* 10
Salad dressing, French *1 tbs* 90
    mayonnaise *1 tbs* 100
Sherbert ½ *cup* 120
Soup, condensed *11 oz can*
    mushroom 360
    noodles 290
    tomato 230
    vegetable 200
Sugar, brown *1 tbs* 50
    granulated *1 tbs* 50
    powdered *1 tbs* 40
Walnuts *8* 100

Drinks

1. Alcohol

    beer *8 oz* 120
    gin *1½ oz* 120
    rum *1½ oz* 150
    whiskey *1½ oz* 150
Wines
    champagne *4 oz* 120
    port *1 oz* 50
    sherry *1 oz* 40
    table, red or white *4 oz* 95

2. Non-alcoholic drinks

Cola, soft drinks, *6 oz bottle* 75
Ginger ale *1 cup* 85
Grapefruit juice, unsweetened *1*
    cup 100
Grape juice ½ *cup* 80
Prune juice ½ *cup* 100
Tomato juice *1 cup* 60

this level. If, on the other hand, you are engaged in strenuous physical exertion at work or recreation, you might need between 2,000 to 3,500 calories a day. It is important to adhere strictly to the allowance, and to do so effectively means it is necessary to weigh the quantities of food you eat.

At first, keeping to a weight-reducing diet is difficult, but with time the body readjusts to the reduced amount of food, and you look back with wonderment at how it was possible to eat so much. It is better to reduce weight gradually by, say, 2 lb (1 kg) a week rather than to indulge in crash diets with rapid weight reduction. Remember it has taken a long time to put on the weight and it will take a considerable time to reduce it.

Salt

Much has been written about the role of salt in high blood pressure (see also page 32), but as yet there is no conclusive proof that it can cause raised blood pressure. Indeed, some studies suggest that it may be of little relevance. Within the medical profession there are two opposing viewpoints on the matter, but the general opinion would seem to be that if you take a lot of salt – and habits vary enormously – and have high blood pressure it would be prudent to cut down your intake, perhaps by not adding salt to your meals at table.

The taste for salt is an acquired one and there seems to be no good reason for encouraging our children to develop a liking for it. In normal conditions our daily salt requirement is provided by our regular diet and by salt added during cooking. There is no need to add more at mealtimes.

The case against it
Studies of primitive populations suggest that in societies which have a low-salt diet high blood pressure is rare. There is some experimental evidence that salt can cause high blood pressure in animals. Diuretic pills which are used in the treatment of high blood pressure exert their effect, at least in part, by increasing the excretion of salt by the kidneys. Dietary restriction of salt has been shown to reduce blood pressure for short periods of time.

So what should you do about salt?
A totally salt-free diet is difficult to achieve, extremely unpleasant and can be dangerous. Our advice to people with high blood pressure who add a lot of salt to their food is to reduce the amount they add by at least 50 per cent, and if possible not to take salt at the table. On the evidence available we believe that for the person with high blood pressure the less salt used the better. You can cut down on the amount you use in cooking by substituting herbs and spices.

The following table shows food with a high salt content and it would be best to avoid or at least cut down on these. You should also consider how foods are prepared, especially in this age of quick-service meals. As one recent review pointed out: 'An order of one of the popular super-burgers, french fries, and a chocolate shake adds up to nearly 1,100 calories. These foods and the condiments added in preparation include 0.540 g of sodium for the hamburger and 0.163 g of sodium on the french fries before the salt is added at the table' which is about the total daily requirement of salt. This underlines the fact that very many prepared and preserved foods contain extremely large amounts of salt. Of preserved foods, only frozen fresh foods are likely to be low in salt.

Foods with high salt content

Biscuits (cookies)	Potato crisps (chips)
Canned vegetables	Pretzels
Ketchup (catsup)	Sardines
Cheese	Sauerkraut
Foods containing self-raising flour	Sausages
Frankfurters	Smoked fish and meat
Ham	Tomato juice (canned)
Pickles	Soya sauce

Cholesterol and fats

Few topics have aroused as much heated controversy in the

correspondence columns of the medical journals as the fat and cholesterol content of the national diet.

A number of fatty substances are transported around the body in the blood stream; some of these are merely part of the general turnover of the fats, or lipids, as they are called medically, that is going on all the time; others come from foods we eat. The liver is the chief regulating organ of fat metabolism, but many organs in the body play an important role. In some cases abnormally high blood-fat levels run in families.

There are two main groups of fat in the food we eat: the saturated fats from animals, which tend to raise the level of cholesterol in the blood, and the polyunsaturated fats from vegetable or marine sources, which do not raise the blood cholesterol. Then there are certain foods which are very high in cholesterol, such as dairy produce, milk, cheese, eggs, butter and shellfish. If we eat a lot of saturated fat and cholesterol-rich foods, particularly with a high calorie content, the level of fats in the blood may rise. Other factors such as obesity, alcohol, the birth control pill and physical inactivity may also increase the blood fats.

If the cholesterol level in the blood is high, this is known medically as hypercholestrolaemia. Another class of fatty substances are triglycerides, which are found in carbohydrates, primarily sugars. A high triglyceride level in the blood is called hypertriglyceridaemia. If levels of some or all the fats in the blood are high, doctors speak of hyperlipidaemia. The fat content of blood can be further classified by measuring the lipoproteins, the substances which transport fats in the blood. Cholesterol is transported by the low-density lipoproteins which tend to be higher when the cholesterol is high.

How these fats contribute to circulatory disease is not completely understood, but it has been suggested that a high consumption of fats in our diet leads to raised levels of lipids in the blood, which may then be deposited in the lining membrane of the arteries, hardening the artery walls and leading to the condition known as atherosclerosis. Furthermore, it is suggested that the high number of people with coronary heart disease in Western society is the result of an excess of fat-rich foods.

Certainly it is true that in the West we eat a lot of these substances, and animal experimentation has shown that cholesterol and saturated fats are associated with atherosclerosis; population studies also show a definite association with high levels of blood cholesterol – hypercholestrolaemia.

However, there is not as yet any firm evidence to prove that reducing the content of cholesterol or fat in the diet will reduce the effects of atherosclerosis – heart attack and stroke – or increase life expectancy.

So what should you do about cholesterol?
Bearing in mind the maxim that we proposed earlier in this book – 'Moderation in all things' – it would not seem unreasonable to apply this to our consumption of fat. There is a substantial amount of evidence linking dietary fat with

---

Low cholesterol foods

Vegetables	Soft margarine	Tea (black)
Fruit	Skimmed milk	Fruit juices
Preserves	Yoghurt	Soft drinks
Cereals	Cottage cheese	Spirits
Flour	Oils (corn,	Wines
Spaghetti	sunflower,olive,	Beers
Biscuits	vegetable)	
(cookies)		

Medium cholesterol foods

White fish	Tuna	Herring
Chicken		

High cholesterol foods

Milk	Cheeses	Meats
Butter	Eggs	Pastry
Margarine	Shellfish	Lard
Cream	Duck	Suet
Ice cream	Goose	

atherosclerosis; and many of us take a diet that is too rich in saturated fat and cholesterol-rich foods. So without going to extremes we could all try to cut down on such foods. By doing so we might do some good.

We should also take animal or saturated fat in moderation by eating lean meat, and grilling rather than frying food; we can use an oil rich in polyunsaturated fat for cooking rather than animal fat. The table on page 63 gives an idea of the cholesterol content of some basic foodstuffs.

Finally, it is worth remembering that we live in the age of synthetic foods, and that our forefathers, who did not suffer from problems of the heart and blood vessels (cardiovascular disease) to anything like the extent that we do, ate a much more natural diet. We might do well ourselves then to revert to more natural foods.

Fibre

The low fibre content of the diets of many Western countries has been blamed for causing or accelerating some bowel and cardiovascular diseases. One recent study has suggested that the lower occurrence of coronary heart disease among people having a high-fibre diet may be due to the fact that their blood pressures are lower than people on a low-fibre diet.

Fibre-rich foods such as cereals, wholemeal bread, potatoes and pulses like beans, peas and lentils need more chewing and fill you up while at the same time adding fewer calories to your daily diet than most people realize. Fibre itself has no calories.

These foods therefore provide a very effective means of slimming without feeling hungry or starved. Remember that it's often the way these foods are cooked that's fattening, not the foods themselves; so try to keep off fried and sugary foods even if they're high in fibre. To find out more about this, read a companion title in this series, *Don't Forget Fibre in Your Diet* by Dr Denis Burkitt (called *Eat Right to Stay Healthy and Enjoy Life More* in North America).

Sugar

There have been suggestions that if you eat a lot of sugar

(sucrose) you run a greater risk of developing arterial disease. The evidence for this claim is not convincing and sugar is no longer considered to be a relevant factor. However, sugar does have a high calorie value and should be taken in moderation if you are trying to lose weight. It is also, of course, bad for your teeth.

Alcohol

There is no evidence that a moderate amount of alcohol does any harm to the cardiovascular system. In fact, there are some indications, admittedly rather tenuous, that alcohol in small amounts may be beneficial. But before you start celebrating, remember that alcoholic drinks do have a high calorie content and when soft drinks are taken as a mix with spirits the calorie content may be considerable. So if you are trying to lose weight you must watch your alcohol consumption.

The position with heavy drinking is quite different. Heavy regular drinking must not be confused with alcoholism, although the recommendations that follow apply to both conditions. Apart from the weight gain that inevitably occurs in heavy drinkers, there are some harmful effects on the heart and circulation. In a recent study in Sweden, heavy alcohol consumption was found to be the single most important factor associated with premature death in middle-aged men. Even a moderate amount of alcohol may elevate your blood pressure, and heavy drinking damages the heart muscle. Another important factor is that heavy drinkers tend to be heavy smokers.

We may, however, take some comfort from the concluding comments of William Kannel from the Framingham Study (see page 18), one of the world's leading experts on risk factors in cardiovascular disease. 'It is encouraging to note that not everything one enjoys in life predisposes to cardiovascular disease. There is nothing to suggest, for the present, that we must give up either coffee or alcohol in moderation to avoid a heart attack. I am sure that many who read this ... will be quite willing to drink to that statement.'

7 ACTIVITY AND EXERCISE

Of all the attempts made by modern society to lead a healthier life, none has been as popular as the craving for physical fitness. Twenty years ago who would have believed it possible to get so many people from both sexes and all age groups running round the streets and parks in track suits. This phenomenon is all the more remarkable in view of the fact that there is no firm evidence to support the popular belief that exercise protects against heart disease and leads to a longer life.

However, there is some evidence, mostly in animals, and to a lesser extent in humans, that exercise may improve the coronary circulation in coronary artery disease. (The coronary arteries, you will remember, are the two arteries that supply blood to the heart muscle.) Also, exercise does appear to lower the cholesterol carrying low-density lipoprotein (lipoproteins are combinations of fats and proteins, see page 62), while increasing the more desirable high-density proportion. Exercise programmes over a period of time can lower blood pressure. In one study there was a mean fall in diastolic blood pressure of nearly 12 mmHg after a six-month controlled exercise programme.

Whatever reservations we may have about the proven value of exercise, there is no doubt that regular exercise and the maintenance of a reasonable state of physical fitness do lead to a general sense of well-being. This beneficial feeling is obviously worth encouraging and it serves as an incentive to adopt a generally healthier lifestyle.

This chapter has been headed 'Activity and exercise' because we want to deal with the subject in two ways. There are many people who would like to take more exercise and become fitter, but who are not prepared to take part in active exercise programmes, or to participate in sporting activities. Some people would not be seen jogging under any circumstances, even if it was guaranteed to prolong life, and many people have disliked sport since school or cannot find one that gives enjoyment. On the other hand, there are those who like jogging, and others who have always been keen on sport. We believe that for those who do not wish to take active exercise it is possible to increase one's daily activity sufficiently to attain a reasonable degree of physical fitness. First let us look at the ways we can do this without committing ourselves to too strict a regimen.

Everyday activity

One of the major problems with modern living is that we have become in many instances almost totally sedentary. It is not uncommon for our daily exertion to consist of no more than walking down the stairs in the morning to the car, and stepping from the car to the office elevator, with a similar energy expenditure in the evening. In former days we would have been obliged to walk or cycle to work.

We have become dependent today on mechanized transport to convey us from one place to another, as if we were invalids. Stand in any supermarket or airport where there is a choice of ordinary stairs or an escalator and note the few, the very few, who will use the former. In office buildings, hospitals and apartment blocks, the ordinary stair has become almost obsolete, a fact that can be judged from the designer's lack of concern with decoration in this area. Everybody uses the elevator. In fact, the stair is often there only because it has to serve as a fire-escape. The person who leads this sedentary existence becomes totally unfit and very often obese. But he could if he wanted increase his daily activity considerably merely by refusing to use the mechanical conveniences of modern life. So, to begin with, you can walk the stairs and refuse to use elevators and escalators. But what of the car?

The car
Again we are hopelessly dependent on this technological convenience. It may be of interest to relate what happens if you try to give up the car.

The first impact is one of inconvenience. We have to use public transport, which is often inefficient. However, after a while this becomes acceptable and one feels a little bit better for the walk to and from the station or bus stop. Then certain other benefits become apparent – it is possible to read the daily paper

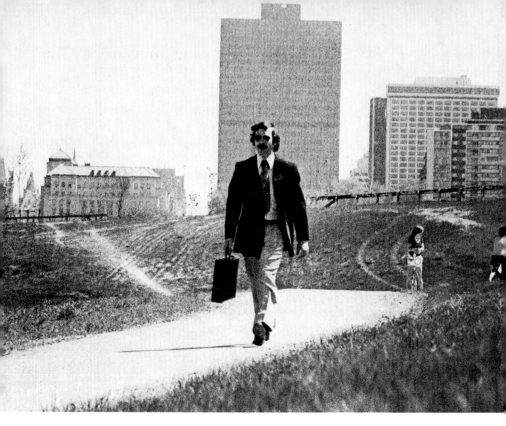

Walking part of the way to work every day is an easy and enjoyable way of building up a reasonable degree of physical fitness.

or a book on the way to and from work. There are the frustrations of breakdowns and delays in the public transport system, but then again cars can also be delayed in rush-hour traffic jams and break down, and there are the increasingly frequent petrol shortages to disrupt private driving.

Then there is the weather. At first this can be sheer misery but after a time you buy suitable clothing. Gradually the concept of distance alters. As a driver you make the most extraordinary efforts to get as close to your destination as possible, often driving round and round and then risking a parking fine. But without the car you walk greater and greater distances, and as this new habit develops distances on foot no longer seem as great as when driving. Soon walking becomes a real pleasure, you take different routes, see places you did not know existed, and meet acquaintances of former years; all in all you feel the better for the experience.

Finally there is the very considerable financial saving: the two-car family can now make do with one car. You are thus contributing actively to the energy conservation principle, and have the satisfaction of helping to keep the environment clean.

Up to now we have spoken of increasing activity in a way that should be within the reach of us all. It calls for a reappraisal of our way of life and an altered approach to our means of moving around. Many of you reading this will be so dependent on the motor car, that you will not believe it possible to make such an apparently drastic change in your way of living. We say to you give it a try, because you will be surprised how much better the alternative is.

Bring back the bike

If we pursue this theme we are brought inevitably to another means of self-propulsion, namely the bicycle. There is no more efficient means of movement than a human on a bicycle. Without utilizing any energy source other than his or her own,

One of the most pleasurable ways to get fit is by cycling – to work, to do the shopping or just for fun!

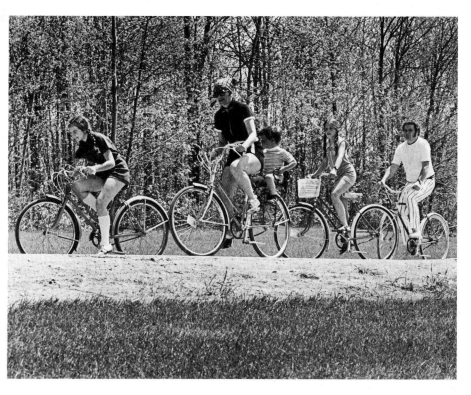

without causing pollution, and with relatively little danger to himself and to others, the cyclist can propel himself along at speeds between 10 and 30 mph (16 and 48 kph) according to his wishes.

The modern bicycle with efficient gears makes cycling one of the most pleasurable of all activities. As a means of going about our daily activities it should be second to none, and indeed it would seem that it will only be a matter of time before it is once again given pride of place. As with cigarette smoking, one can only view with dismay the impotence of governments, which on the one hand advocate energy conservation and environmental purity, and on the other do nothing to encourage the return of the cyclist to the roads. Admittedly, some countries have shown greater wisdom in the matter by providing cycle lanes, cycle parks and adequate training facilities for children; while others have shown an almost total lack of realism in providing the necessary facilities for a population that is once again willing to take to the roads on two wheels.

You will, of course, have to contend with the vagaries of weather but, as with walking, thanks to the development of new synthetic waterproof clothing, this drawback can be overcome, but make sure you wear colours that can be easily seen. 'Bring back the bike' is no longer a plaintive cry from a few, it is developing its own popular momentum as can be seen by increasing bicycle sales.

Exercise

Jogging, calisthenic exercises, and games such as golf, squash, tennis, or whatever one likes, all have their place according to what suits the individual. There is, however, one cardinal principle underlying all sporting activities and exercise, and that is: if you have been leading a sedentary existence and are now planning to become more active, return to activity gradually and cautiously.

There is no reason why you cannot achieve peak fitness for your age at any time in your life, but the older you get the more cautious you have to be. If, for example, you are in your mid-forties and decide that having once played squash you would now like to take up the sport again there is probably no reason why you should not do so. But it might be prudent to have a

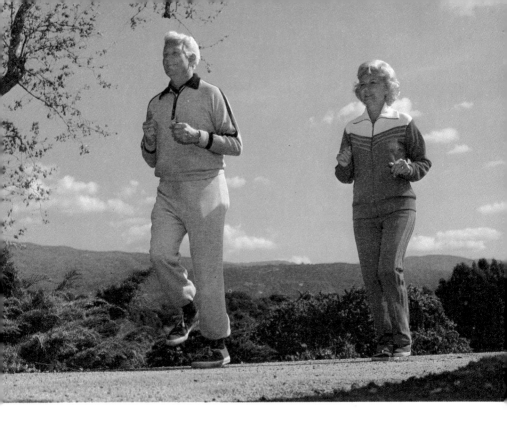

If you intend to take up a new sporting activity such as jogging, it is important to take it easy at first.

physical check-up first. Then you should find someone else of your own age anxious to take up the game, and begin gently. After a few weeks you can move onto more competitive partners providing you do not try to out-do each other in competitiveness.

Don't force the pace

A word of caution: if you overdo exercise after a long period of inactivity you can get arthritis, injuries to the tendons or, at the very least, stiff muscles. More recently, stress fractures of various bones in the legs and pelvis have been associated with jogging. So whatever activity you take up do return to it gradually. And bear in mind that you will probably get more benefit out of the exercise as well as be more inclined to keep it up, if you take up something you enjoy doing.

Sex and high blood pressure

Blood pressure and heart rate increase during sexual intercourse, sometimes dramatically, even in people with normal blood pressure. However, this does not mean that people with high blood pressure have to give up sex. It is not possible here to lay down general recommendations about sexual activity for people with high blood pressure, a talk with your doctor is the best way to clarify the situation. If your blood pressure is poorly controlled it would be advisable to refrain from excessive sexual activity until your doctor is satisfied that your condition is improving.

If you notice that your sexual performance is deteriorating, it could be that one of the antihypertensive drugs you may be taking is at least partially responsible. Modern drugs do not usually affect sexual performance, but it is worth mentioning it to your doctor should the problem occur.

Is a change of lifestyle worth while?

In the last decade there has been a dramatic decline – over 20 per cent – in coronary heart disease and stroke in North America. This remarkable change has coincided with a striking change in lifestyle. Is it coincidence, or cause and effect? The answer is not known, but there are some pointers.

In North Karelia in Finland a five-year community programme designed to reduce smoking, cholesterol and blood pressure in a population of 10,000 brought a reduction in the estimated risk of coronary heart disease of 17 per cent among men and 12 per cent among women. Furthermore, there was an overall decrease in the death rate of 5 per cent. Deaths from cardio-vascular disease decreased by 13 per cent among men and 31 per cent among women aged between thirty and sixty-four years.

On the basis of such figures it does seem to make good sense to observe the advice recommended in this chapter (and in chapters five and six): take regular exercise, don't drive when you can walk, and every so often try using the stairs instead of the elevator.

It is not possible unfortunately, to give such categorical advice about another aspect of our lives which is also considered a risk factor for those with high blood pressure, namely, stress.

8 THE ROLE OF STRESS

There is a popular belief that stress is a major cause of high blood pressure. Indeed the word 'hypertension', which means high blood pressure, tends to suggest this. The evidence, however, is far from convincing. Stress is extremely difficult to define and almost impossible to measure, so it is very hard to prove a cause-and-effect relationship between high blood pressure and stress.

It has been argued that one of the causes of the great increase in coronary artery disease and high blood pressure in this century has been the increased stress of life, particularly urban life. However, it could equally be argued that the stresses of survival of former times were, if anything, greater than they are today. Whatever the answer, the conclusion for those of us wishing to lead a healthier life must be that too much stress is not a good thing. We know this from the unpleasant effects of excessive stress on the mind and body generally: we become irritable, may not sleep well, have tension headaches, and we may develop a number of so-called psychosomatic symptoms, such as a rapid heart rate with palpitations, bowel upsets and so on.

Of course, a certain amount of stress is essential for the drive and competition that is so much a part of life. Ideally our lives should be planned so that we have an adequate amount of work, and sufficient time for relaxation. But all too often work spills over into play, leaving insufficient time for relaxing.

Acute stress may occasionally precipitate a heart attack in susceptible people and blood pressure certainly rises in response to stress, but it is difficult to prove exactly to what extent stress is a factor. Perhaps we should be guided by the Joint Working Party of the Royal College of Physicians of London and the British Cardiac Society: 'Initiative, diligence, leadership and hard work, especially in young people, should not be discouraged on the mistaken supposition that these qualities are indicative of future coronary heart disease.'

Personality type

Many of the stresses of life are to a certain extent self-inflicted, or at least so it would seem to some. For example, the placid unambitious member of the work-team, who enjoys his weekends fishing, reading, golfing or whatever, finds it difficult to understand the mentality of his aggressive ambitious colleague who has little time for family or recreational activity. The latter in turn finds his colleague's lack of drive somewhat frustrating, although he may begrudgingly admire his ability to relax and enjoy himself.

Personalities have been classified into two groups: Type A and Type B. Type A is the dynamic, driving, aggressive and ambitious individual who is preoccupied with time and deadlines; whereas the Type B personality is easy-going, has little regard for time, may not seek to get to the top, and although his competitive drive is less, he may ironically get further than his Type A counterpart by virtue of the fact that he just lives longer. Type A personalities are said to have twice the risk of coronary heart disease of their Type B colleagues, but both types are susceptible to high blood pressure as the two following case histories show. The first example describes a fairly typical Type A personality.

Mr Victor Speed is president of a large merchant-banking company. He was appointed to this post when aged only forty-two. From the moment he left school he seemed to waste no time in getting to the top. After leaving university with an honours degree he worked with a number of companies before joining the banking concern of which is he now the head. His colleagues respected him but few had ever got really to know him. He had a reputation for being fair, and it was said that he could be ruthless if an issue barred his progress.

He gave himself totally to his work and demanded the same from his colleagues, many of whom over the years found the pace intolerable and departed to more peaceful jobs. He was obsessional about time and could not tolerate unpunctuality or failure to meet a deadline. It was rumoured that he wore two watches. His family life was said to be none too happy. As he travelled frequently and always brought home work from the office, which he rarely left before 7 pm, there was little time for relaxation with his family. Business meetings and dinners often kept him late in the evenings.

It came as little surprise to his colleagues when it was announced that he had had a heart attack in Hong Kong. When he returned to the office some months later he delegated much of his work to the vice-president and it was noted that he no longer smoked and that he took every second afternoon off for a game of golf. Everyone relaxed a little.

But the easy-going type who never seems to worry about time or climbing the promotional ladder may also have high blood pressure. Mr Joe Slocum is an assistant secretary in government service, a post he has occupied for fifteen years. In that time he has seen younger men appointed to more senior posts, and he is aware that many of his junior colleagues consider that if he were more aggressive in his dealings with the head of his department he would have been a first secretary by now. Another source of annoyance to these junior colleagues who have a very high regard and no small measure of affection for their boss is the knowledge that Mr Slocum's immediate superior presents to the head of his department as his own work the work done by Mr Slocum. But then Mr Slocum doesn't seem to mind. Besides, he has so many other interests, one of which – the collection of books on his native city – tends to distract him so during the lunch-break (when he browses in the bookshops) that he is often at a loss to explain how he could have mistaken the hour.

On such occasions all the clerks and typists wink knowingly as Mr Slocum produces an old gold watch on a chain from his waistcoat pocket and staring over his spectacles at the office clock makes intricate adjustments to his chronometer which all present know has not worked for some thirty years.

For many years it had been Mr Slocum's practice to have two or three beers with a few of his colleagues each evening before returning home. They were disappointed to find recently that he could no longer join them, as his doctor had instructed him to lose weight on account of his high blood pressure.

Should we change the way we live?

In general, those with high blood pressure should try to avoid undue stress and to take time off for rest and relaxation. Some people may be helped by learning one of the relaxation techniques which have received more and more attention in recent years.

Ways to relax

Yoga   This term is a collective one for many variant Hindu meditative practices which are often combined with physical exercises involving control of posture and breathing.

Some studies have shown a considerable improvement in people with high blood pressure who have been practising yoga, especially among those using the method of Chandra Patel, which combines a form of yoga with biofeedback (see below). Of all behavioural techniques, this is the best researched, and the one that for the present holds the greatest promise.

Transcendental meditation (TM)   In this form of meditation relaxation is achieved by thinking of a word or sound (mantra) and, as it were, switching off from the external world. Once the technique has been acquired it can be practised a few times daily.

In a number of studies a significant fall in blood pressure has been achieved, but the long-term value of the method has not been established.

Progressive muscle relaxation (PMR)   The purpose of this technique is to achieve conscious control over muscle groups and to induce a low level of generalized muscle tone for the purpose of controlling anxiety. In a quiet setting the subject is placed in a comfortable position and is instructed to systematically tense and relax various muscles.

Most research with PMR has been in the treatment of phobias, but some studies have shown a promising reduction in blood pressure.

Biofeedback   Certain functions such as heart rate, blood pressure and skin temperature are controlled without conscious awareness. For example, our heart rate changes frequently during the day according to the needs of our bodies, but we are usually unaware of this. The control mechanism is involuntary, as distinct from a voluntary process such as walking.

The principle in biofeedback is that the subject is informed by electromechanical devices about change of, say, blood pressure

76

on a second-by-second or minute-by-minute basis. Then the subject attempts to control the blood pressure level according to the information fed back by the machine, the process often being reinforced by rewards when success is achieved. In short, the person is trained to exercise some control over these involuntary processes.

In a recent review of the subject it was concluded that blood pressure could be reduced significantly during biofeedback training. The reduction was small in people with normal pressures, but there was a significant reduction in both systolic and diastolic values in subjects with high blood pressure.

Although biofeedback may be an effective means of lowering blood pressure at a given session, the sustained effect of reducing blood pressure with home practice has not been conclusively demonstrated and it is on this long-term result that the success of the technique will ultimately be judged. A great deal more research is needed.

Hypnosis   On its own, hypnosis does not alter blood pressure. There is some evidence that if it is used together with other relaxation techniques the blood pressure can be reduced, but as yet the value of hypnosis has not been assessed.

There are many variations of the meditation/relaxation concept, all of which attempt to modify physiological functions such as blood pressure. In common with most behavioural techniques they have not been fully evaluated, but a careful study of the literature suggests that it is indeed possible in the short term to reduce blood pressure with biofeedback and relaxation techniques. A combination of both methods is perhaps the most effective.

The long-term benefit of these techniques is only now being investigated. It would seem that daily practice will be necessary and this raises the question as to whether people will be prepared to stick to the routine on a more or less permanent basis. The same problem applies of course to drug treatment, and however sceptical we may be of the scientific validity of some of the studies so far carried out on these techniques, there seems to be one common factor – you feel better afterwards.

A companion title in this series, *Stress and Relaxation* by Jane Madders, provides a useful introduction to self-help methods of relaxation.

9 WOMEN AND HIGH BLOOD PRESSURE

There is some evidence that women react differently from men to high blood pressure. Among young adults high blood pressure occurs more frequently in men. Between the ages of twenty-five and thirty-five, 21 per cent of men have a diastolic pressure greater than 90 mmHg, whereas only 9 per cent of women have blood pressure of this magnitude or more. With increasing age the difference between the sexes becomes less and between the ages of fifty-five and sixty-four, about 40 per

This shows the changes in systolic and diastolic pressure in men and women as they get older. Systolic pressure keeps rising but diastolic pressure, particularly in men, levels off.

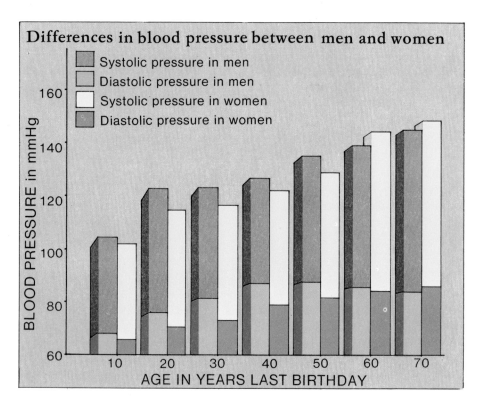

Differences in blood pressure between men and women

- Systolic pressure in men
- Diastolic pressure in men
- Systolic pressure in women
- Diastolic pressure in women

BLOOD PRESSURE in mmHg

AGE IN YEARS LAST BIRTHDAY

cent of both men and women have diastolic pressures higher than 90 mmHg.

Women appear to tolerate high blood pressure better than men, and the death rate from the complications of high blood pressure is higher for men than for women.

However, high blood pressure can cause special problems among women. During their reproductive years there are the problems of high blood pressure in pregnancy and toxaemia, a condition in which there is salt and water retention, protein in the urine, and swelling of the ankles and fingers. Furthermore, high blood pressure in some women is caused, or aggravated, by the birth control pill.

The pill and high blood pressure

Almost all women taking oral contraceptives containing the hormone oestrogen have a rise in blood pressure. This rise is usually only slight and generally does not bring the blood pressure into the high or abnormal range. However, about 4 per cent of women on the pill do develop diastolic pressures of 90 mmHg or greater. Put another way, this means that twice as many women on the pill will have this level of blood pressure as compared to women not taking the pill. In fact, high blood pressure caused by the pill is probably the commonest type of blood pressure with an identifiable cause.

The exact way in which the pill causes high blood pressure is not known. It may be that the hormones interfere with the renin mechanism (see page 16) and cause salt retention. The oestrogen component of the pill is considered to be the hormone responsible for the rise in blood pressure, and most contraceptive pills now contain only a low dose of oestrogen combined with progesterone; some are available containing progesterone only. It is not yet known for sure whether either of these types will cause less high blood pressure.

Unfortunately, there is no way of telling which women will develop high blood pressure on the pill, but there is some evidence to suggest that women who have had toxaemia or high blood pressure during pregnancy may develop pill-induced high blood pressure. This group, and women who already have high blood pressure or who have kidney disease, should avoid oral contraceptives if possible.

The long-term effects of high blood pressure brought on by the pill are largely unknown. Women who have taken the pill seem to have an increased risk of developing heart attack or stroke, but this is not necessarily because of the high blood pressure. Once the pill is stopped pressure usually returns to normal, although it may take a month or so for this to happen.

A rise in blood pressure is more likely among older women taking the pill and among those taking it over a long period. Studies have shown that most of the cardiovascular deaths among women on the pill occur in women over thirty-five who have been using the pill for a long time and who smoke.

What should you do?
If you are thinking of going on the pill, there are a few points you should consider first. It would be as well to look at alternative forms of contraception if you are over thirty-five, if you are over thirty and smoke, of if you have a history of clotting disorders (such as thrombosis or embolism), stroke, heart disease or high blood pressure. You should never start the pill without going to your doctor and having a full examination. A record will then be made of your personal and family history, and a full clinical examination taken, including measurement of your blood pressure and weight, a breast and pelvic examination and a cervical smear. The result of this initial examination, and subsequent ones, should be entered on a special record card. You will be asked either to retain this and bring it to each follow-up visit, or the doctor or clinic will keep it for you.

You should be re-examined three months after starting the pill and thereafter at six-monthly intervals, with special attention being paid to your blood pressure.

What happens if you develop high blood pressure?
If your blood pressure rises to or above 150/90 mmHg your doctor will advise you to stop taking the pill, probably for at least three months. Usually the blood pressure will return to normal in about this time and then it is reasonable to assume that the pill was the cause of the rise and an alternative contraceptive method should be used. If the blood pressure is not back to normal after three months, it becomes more difficult to implicate the pill as the cause of the rise. Nevertheless, we believe that another form of contraceptive should be used in such cases. Observation can be continued for another six

months if the rise in blood pressure is not severe, or treatment of the high blood pressure may be called for.

The important points to remember are that the pill has a number of potential dangers, but that for the great majority of women it does not cause any problems. However, it is only by looking carefully for those problems which are likely to arise that doctors can prevent the possible dangers. Always have your regular check-up if you are taking the pill, and in particular make sure that your blood pressure is measured at each attendance.

Pregnancy and high blood pressure

High blood pressure in pregnancy calls for careful supervision because the doctor has to consider the risks to both the mother and the unborn child. Most women with mild elevation of blood pressure do very well when they are pregnant, and high blood pressure in itself is not a reason for avoiding pregnancy. In fact, the effect of pregnancy on women whose blood pressure is already high is quite unpredictable. In one-third there will be no change, in another third there will be an increase, and in the remaining third the blood pressure will fall to normal or below normal during pregnancy.

Providing you see your doctor regularly and follow his advice during your pregnancy there is no reason if you have mild high blood pressure why delivery should not be perfectly normal.

When the blood pressure is high during pregnancy the doctor has to consider three possibilities: the pregnancy itself may have raised the blood pressure; it may have brought to light pre-existing high blood pressure that had not been diagnosed; or the rise in blood pressure may be caused by toxaemia of pregnancy which, as we have seen (page 79), is a more serious condition. Toxaemia of pregnancy (sometimes called eclampsia or pre-eclamptic toxaemia) can endanger the mother's life and that of the unborn child and it is usually best for the woman to have treatment in hospital. In some cases labour may have to be induced and a Caesarian section performed. After the baby is born the blood pressure usually returns to normal.

High blood pressure in pregnancy that is not caused by toxaemia can be treated in much the same way as high blood pressure in non-pregnant women, but there are some important differences. For example, detailed investigation will be deferred until after the birth of the baby. This is particularly important in the case of X-ray examinations which can be harmful to the developing foetus. Also, the unborn child could be affected by any drugs which the mother takes. Drugs can cross the placental barrier and with some drugs this can lead to malformations. Because the effect on the foetus is unknown, doctors try to prescribe as few drugs as possible during pregnancy, and to use only those which are known to be safe. Therefore, when treating high blood pressure, the first approach will be to see whether it can be lowered by weight reduction and salt restriction.

Thiazide diuretics, drugs which gradually reduce body fluid and thus blood pressure (see page 88), have been shown to be safe in pregnancy, but they do raise the level of a substance in the blood called urate which is an indicator of the maturity of the developing foetus. Some obstetricians, therefore, prefer

Regular blood pressure checks are especially important during pregnancy.

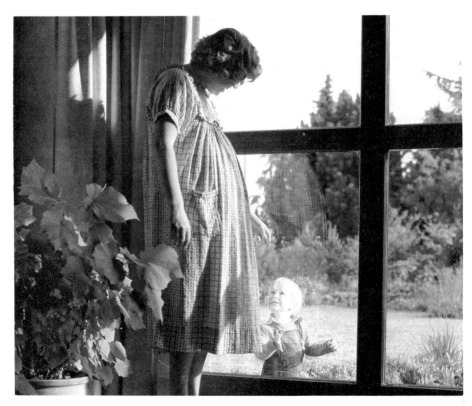

not to use these drugs. Methyldopa (trade name Aldomet) and hydralazine (trade name Apresoline) have also been shown to be safe, and a limited number of studies suggest that drugs which slow the heart called beta-blockers – at least, the older ones such as propranolol (trade name Inderal) – do not harm the unborn child. For a fuller discussion of these see the next chapter.

It is very important if you are taking drugs for your high blood pressure and find that you are pregnant to ask your doctor whether the drug could be harmful to the baby. If you have been on drugs for high blood pressure for a long time, you should let your doctor know at the earliest moment about your pregnancy so that he can advise on the best treatment for you and your baby. Unfortunately, it does happen that people get so used to taking their blood-pressure-lowering drugs that they forget to mention them when they attend the ante-natal clinic. Remember then to tell your doctor or the clinic as soon as possible.

With modern treatment even very severe cases of high blood pressure can be brought through pregnancy safely. But if you do have problems during pregnancy because of your high blood pressure it would be as well to discuss the advisability of having more children with your family doctor and obstetrician.

Obesity in pregnancy
Obesity is associated with high blood pressure in pregnancy (but not with toxaemia), so you should try to keep to the ideal weight throughout your pregnancy.

Hormone replacement therapy

The oestrogen hormone is now being used increasingly for hormone replacement therapy for women during the menopause. It seems likely that in the future it may be as widely used for menopausal symptoms as for oral contraception. As yet there is not enough evidence to say how safe this form of treatment will prove to be. However, as with the pill, we can anticipate that hormone replacement therapy will increase the risk of some cardiovascular disorders for at least certain women. It is therefore advisable for women who are considering this form of therapy to have a full examination before starting treatment and to attend regularly for check-ups and especially measurement of blood pressure, for, like the pill, hormone replacement therapy can cause a rise in blood pressure.

10 DRUG TREATMENT

The availability of effective drugs has revolutionized the treatment of high blood pressure in the last quarter of a century. The first effective drugs to lower high blood pressure were used in the late 1940s and early 1950s. Compared with modern drugs these were extremely crude. Although they were effective in lowering blood pressure, their use was associated with very unpleasant side-effects in most patients to whom they were given. Furthermore, in those early days most of these drugs had to be given by injection. Not surprisingly, use was restricted to the more severe cases of high blood pressure.

Today there are many drugs from which the doctor can choose. These drugs are extremely effective in lowering blood pressure, but as with all potent medicines unwanted side-effects do occur and must be watched for. However, when wisely used the number of such effects is low. It may take a period of trial and error to find the drug that is both effective and free of troublesome side-effects for each individual. In addition, the dose may have to be changed because people differ in their response to drugs. What suits one person may not suit another. This process normally takes four to five visits to your doctor, though with some people the first drug and the initial dose may be satisfactory, so subsequent visits can be spaced more widely. With other people it may be very difficult indeed to select the most suitable drug or combination of drugs. Thus, finding the right drug treatment may be time-consuming, but in the end it is time well spent. Moreover, with most people the response to treatment is quick. Difficulties, if there are any, occur most often among people who have severe high blood pressure.

General approach

Irrespective of whether or not drug treatment will be required your doctor will always advise you to change your lifestyle if he thinks this is necessary. In chapters five, six and seven we have discussed the advantages of stopping smoking, taking care of your diet, reducing weight, and taking regular exercise. However, some people, although they might follow their doctor's advice on these matters to the letter, still have high blood pressure and for them drug treatment must be considered. In other words, for people whose diastolic blood pressure is consistently above 100 mmHg and who have failed to respond to the general measures outlined earlier, drug treatment may be the only answer. As already discussed, the value of blood-pressure-lowering drugs is not so well established with pressures in the 90–100 mmHg range. However, when the doctor weighs up all the relevant factors he may well decide to prescribe drugs for people whose blood pressure is within this range.

Because the drug treatment of high blood pressure is usually lifelong the decision to start treatment is an extremely important one.

Is there an ideal drug?

The ideal drug should have the following characteristics: it should be effective in controlling blood pressure throughout the twenty-four hours of the day when given in one, or at most two, doses per day; it should control the various increases in blood pressure that are liable to occur at certain times of the day, and also the sudden surges associated with exertion and strenuous exercise; it should have no unwanted side-effects; it should be inexpensive; and finally, it should be easy to find the correct dose for each individual.

Because of the great strides made by the pharmaceutical industry in the past two decades, many of the drugs used today for the treatment of high blood pressure are not far short of these ideals.

What are the drugs used today?

Drugs used to lower high blood pressure are called antihypertensive drugs or antihypertensives. The number and kind available vary somewhat from country to country because the drug regulatory agencies set up by the various nations differ in their selection of the drugs that can be put on sale. In most Western countries there are at least fifty different drugs or drug combinations used in the treatment of high blood pressure. It would clearly be impractical to list them all and we have not attempted to be comprehensive, but several representative examples are mentioned.

It is easier to understand these drugs if we classify them into four main groups as follows:

1. Diuretics, which decrease fluid and salt in the circulation.
2. Beta adrenoceptor blocking drugs (generally shortened to 'beta-blockers'), which slow the heart.
3. Vasodilators, which widen the blood vessels.
4. Drugs acting on the nervous system.

Diuretics act on the kidneys. Vasodilators relax blood vessels. The main action of beta-blockers is to slow the heart. Drugs acting on the nervous system affect the brain and the ends of the sympathetic nerves.

Sites of action of blood-pressure-lowering drugs

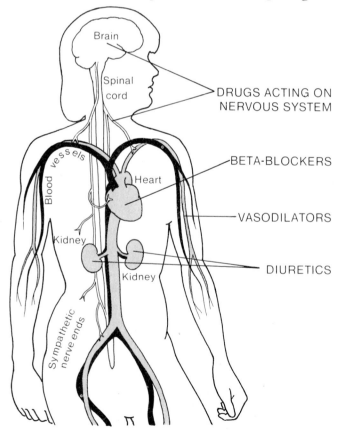

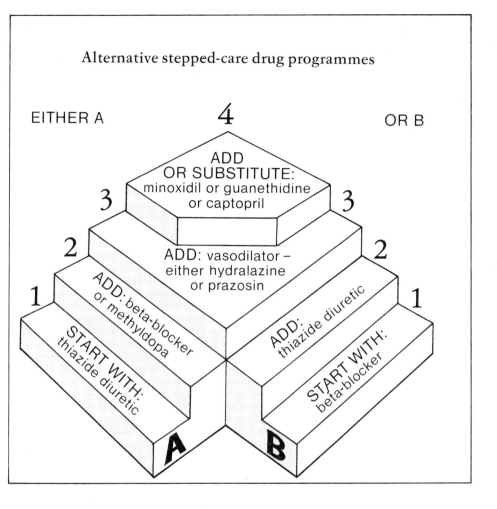

Alternative stepped-care drug programmes

EITHER A   4   OR B

ADD OR SUBSTITUTE: minoxidil or guanethidine or captopril

ADD: vasodilator – either hydralazine or prazosin

ADD: beta-blocker or methyldopa

ADD: thiazide diuretic

START WITH: thiazide diuretic

START WITH: beta-blocker

A   B

Depending on the patient's circumstances the doctor might recommend either programme A or B. Failure to control blood pressure leads to the next step. It is most often controlled at step 2. Steps 2 and 3 in B are sometimes reversed.

To begin with your doctor will probably select either a beta-blocker or a diuretic. He will start with a low dose of a beta-blocker, or a standard dose of diuretic, and at regular intervals he will measure your blood pressure and watch for any unwanted side-effects. You can help by letting him know how you feel. We will be mentioning some of the more common side-effects, but if you notice something else unusual do not hesitate to tell your doctor as it could be due to the drug.

In the so-called 'stepped care' system recommended by the World Health Organization, a diuretic or beta-blocker may be used as the first step in initial therapy. If this is not effective in controlling the blood pressure, the doctor moves to the second step in which these drugs may be combined with each other, or one or other of them may be combined with some other blood-pressure-lowering drug. On the rare occasion when blood pressure does not respond adequately to such a regimen the third or fourth step may be taken when various combinations of drugs can be employed. People with very resistant high blood pressure may also be offered newer drugs, some of which have only recently come on the market. Some in fact are so new that they are not available for general use. These are generally only used by doctors working within the hospital framework. In any event your doctor will explain the pros and cons of using drugs that are still in the research stage.

Oddly enough, you may feel less well when you first start your drugs. Common symptoms are tiredness and lack of energy. This can happen when the blood pressure is lowered after a period of prolonged elevation. It seems to take some time for the circulation and the metabolism to get accustomed to the lower pressure, but after some weeks your previous state of well-being should return.

Diuretics

A diuretic may be defined as a drug that increases the amount of salt and water excreted by the kidney each day. This is, of course, reflected by the amount of urine passed each day. Diuretics have been used for the treatment of high blood pressure since the early 1960s. For many physicians they are the first choice in drugs when treatment has to be started.

How do they work?
By increasing salt and water excretion the diuretic decreases the amount of fluid in the circulation. This has the effect of lowering the blood pressure. It is also thought that the diuretic lowers blood pressure by decreasing the amount of fluid contained in the actual cells of the blood vessel wall. The vessels thus become less resistant to the blood.

Diuretics are effective in controlling mild and even moderate elevation of blood pressure, and can be given alone for this purpose. Severe high blood pressure generally does not respond to a diuretic as sole treatment. However, as mild high blood pressure is much the most common form, a good result can be confidently expected for most people who begin with diuretics. The blood-pressure-lowering effect of the diuretic lasts throughout the day and as a group they are inexpensive – two important characteristics of our ideal drug.

Possible unwanted effects
Diuretics all produce some unwanted side-effects. Most of these changes occur at the chemical level in the body.

Elevated blood sugar   The amount of sugar in the blood is frequently raised in people who are taking diuretics, but only in a small number of cases does this present a problem. The increase in sugar can be detected by measuring the amount of glucose in the blood. If the blood sugar is above a certain level, it appears in the urine and can be detected quite easily. With someone who is susceptible to diabetes a diuretic may unmask the condition. In general, therefore, we try to avoid the use of diuretics in people who have diabetes.

Potassium loss   By their action on the kidney, diuretics tend to cause some loss of potassium. Potassium is a salt very like sodium – sodium chloride is common table salt – which must be present in the correct amount for proper functioning of the body. There are a number of ways of dealing with potassium loss. Some doctors prescribe pills which contain potassium in addition to the diuretic. These diuretics have the letter K, which is the chemical formula for potassium, added to the trade name of the drug, for example Centyl K, Esidrex K. (The trade name of a drug is the name given to the particular preparation by the company that manufactures it; the approved or generic name is the name which has the approval of the relevant government agency or department.) Often this diuretic-potassium combination is prescribed when drug treatment is first started so as to prevent a gradual loss of potassium from the body. However, it should be noted that potassium loss leads to problems in only a very small number of people, perhaps about 5 per cent.

A second way of counteracting potassium loss is to combine a potassium-losing diuretic with a potassium-conserving one. However, while these have the desired effect of keeping potassium levels within the normal range, they are a good deal more expensive. Since only a few people develop a deficiency in potassium in the normal course of events, it is probably not necessary to give potassium tablets to otherwise healthy young and middle-aged people with high blood pressure, although for the elderly and for those taking other drugs it may be wise to do so.

The healthiest way to supplement the intake of potassium in the diet is to eat more of the foods which are rich in potassium, for example, bananas, oranges – in fact, most fresh fruits. In addition, many fresh vegetables contain good supplies of potassium.

Potassium-rich foods

Fresh fruits	Fresh vegetables
Apples	Asparagus
Apricots	Beans
Avocado	Brussels sprouts
Banana	Cabbage
Dates	Corn on the cob
Grapefruit (and juice)	Peas
Oranges (and juice)	Peppers
Prunes	*Potatoes*
Raisins	Radishes

(Foods in italics are especially helpful)

Gout Uric acid is the chemical involved in gout, a painful condition of the joints which picks out the big toe in particular. Diuretics may cause an increase in uric acid in the body and in rare instances may trigger an attack of gout. Therefore we avoid prescribing diuretics for people who have gout.

Excessive loss of fluid If diuretics are taken in large doses, or if the person taking them is particularly sensitive to their action, dehydration may occur – that is, the diuretic may cause an excessive loss of fluid. This is unusual. Early signs of excessive fluid loss are a feeling of dizziness on standing and dryness of the mouth. Usually, once the diuretic has been stopped the condition improves.

Which diuretic is best?
There are two groups of diuretics used in the treatment of high

Diuretic drugs used to lower blood pressure

Approved name	UK trade name	US trade name	Canadian trade name	Australian trade name
THIAZIDES: bendrofluazide (UK, Australia) bendroflumethiazide (US, Canada)	Centyl†	Naturetin	Naturetin†	Pluryl
chlorothiazide	Saluric	Diuril	Diuril	Chlotride
chlorthalidone	Hygroton†	Hygroton	Hygroton	Hygroton
clopamide	Brinaldix†			Brinaldix
cyclopenthiazide	Navidrex†			Navidrex
hydrochlorothiazide	Esidrex†	Esidrix	Esidrix†	Esidrex
methyclothiazide	Enduron	Enduron	Diuretic	Enduron
metolazone	Metenix	Zaroxolyn	Zaroxolyn	Diulo
polythiazide	Nephril	Renese	Renese	
'LOOP' DIURETICS: bumetanide	Burinex†			
ethacrynic acid	Edecrin	Edecrin	Edecrin	Edecril
frusemide (UK, Australia) furosemide (US, Canada)	Lasix† Diumide-K*	Lasix	Lasix	Lasix

† preparations available with potassium added
* only available as a combination preparation: frusemide and potassium

blood pressure: thiazides and 'loop' diuretics. How do they compare? The thiazides have a longer action on the kidney so that the increased amount of urine may be passed unnoticed by the person taking them. They produce their effect gradually and gently.

With the 'loop' diuretic the story is different. Here the effect of the drug is quite rapid in onset and a large volume of urine may be passed within a few hours of taking the pill and this may be uncomfortable and inconvenient. Most of this effect is over in three or four hours. The tendency of the two groups of diuretics to cause the chemical problems discussed above is roughly equal. Finally, it should be said that the 'loop' diuretics usually cost more than most thiazide diuretics. For these reasons the thiazides are preferred in the treatment of high blood pressure.

Beta-blockers

More precisely these drugs should be termed beta adrenoceptor blocking drugs, but in practice doctors usually call them 'beta-blockers'. In 1966 as a result of the pioneering work of Dr Brian Prichard propranolol (trade name Inderal) was introduced and since then at least another nine beta-blockers have been made available for the treatment of high blood pressure. The precise number available varies slightly from country to country. Their introduction into Britain and Australia in 1966 was a major landmark in high blood pressure treatment. They were introduced into Canada two years later.

What they do

The actions of these drugs on the circulation are quite complex and from a theoretical standpoint the drug has one property which one might have predicted would lead to an increase in blood pressure rather than a fall. Because of this, some time elapsed before Dr Prichard's findings were introduced to clinical practice. Indeed, resistance to the introduction of this drug in the United States meant that Inderal was only made available there for the treatment of high blood pressure as recently as 1976. Since then two additional drugs belonging to

Beta-blocker drugs used to lower blood pressure

Approved name	UK trade name	US trade name	Canadian trade name	Australian trade name
acebutolol*	Sectral			
atenolol*	Tenormin			Tenormin
labetalol	Trandate			Trandate
metoprolol*	{ Betaloc		Betaloc	Betaloc
	Lopressor	Lopressor	Lopressor	Lopressor
nadolol	Corgard	Corgard	Corgard	
oxprenolol	Trasicor		Trasicor	Trasicor
pindolol	Visken		Visken	Visken
propranolol	Inderal	Inderal	Inderal	Inderal
sotalol	Sotacor			
timolol	{ Betim		Blocadren	Blocadren
	Blocadren			

* selective action (see text)

this group have come on the market in the United States. Beta-blockers are now used on a large scale in most countries in the world.

They are quite effective in lowering blood pressure, particularly among young people with high blood pressure. They have a smooth action and rarely, if ever, cause excessive fall in blood pressure. To some extent they prevent the surges in blood pressure that occur with emotion and exertion. They are all effective in keeping control throughout the twenty-four hours of the day when taken as a single dose. However, while many drugs in this group are reasonably priced they are more expensive than diuretics. The cheapest beta-blockers are close in price to the most expensive diuretics, but the most expensive beta-blockers are quite costly. Again it should be emphasized that although price is important there are other factors to be taken into account in making the choice of drugs. It is only when all other things are equal that the price should become the deciding factor.

Possible unwanted effects

Beta-blockers reduce many of the actions of adrenaline (epinephrine) on the circulation and many other parts of the body. These effects are often apparent to the person taking the drug. Normally the rate at which the heart beats is determined by the level of adrenaline in the blood and as these drugs counteract the action of adrenaline they consequently lower the pulse rate. And because beta-blockers counteract the action of adrenaline on the heart, occasionally when there is heart disease the pumping action of the heart is reduced and what is known as 'heart failure' may occur. In heart failure, the heart continues to pump blood but not as efficiently as before.

Adrenaline also helps to keep the air passages (bronchi) wide so as to allow air into and out of the lungs. In some susceptible people beta-blockers block this action and thereby cause the person to wheeze. This is most likely in asthmatics, but wheezing may sometimes occur in people who have not previously complained of any respiratory problems. Therefore, we would not advise the use of beta-blockers for asthmatics.

Some of the new beta-blockers are selective in their action and their main effect is on the heart. When taken in low doses they have little or no effect on the air passages. These drugs are useful for people with bronchitis, but for asthmatics all beta-blockers are best avoided. One of the commonest problems that people who are taking beta-blockers notice is that their hands and feet get cold. This happens most often in winter, but it can also happen in summer or when the weather is quite mild. The selective blockers don't seem to cause this problem as frequently as others, but the evidence on this is not complete.

Other possible unwanted side-effects include vivid dreams, depression and sleep disturbances. This is because some of the beta-blockers gain access to the brain. All these effects can be reversed by stopping the drug, or on occasion your doctor may decide simply to reduce the dose so as to minimize the problem.

You may think from what we have said that beta-blockers sound dangerous, but when they are used properly the number of unwanted side-effects is very low indeed. They are given for many conditions in addition to high blood pressure. Perhaps their commonest use is in the treatment of angina, or, to give it its full name, angina pectoris. This is chest pain associated with narrowing of the coronary arteries. If someone has both high blood pressure and angina the use of a beta-blocker is particularly appropriate. However, the decision to prescribe this drug, or indeed any other drugs, must take into account any factors which indicate against its use.

Vasodilators

How they work
There are many nervous, hormonal and chemical factors that influence the circulation and control the level of blood pressure. The final common pathway for these forces is the blood vessels themselves. It is changes in these vessels that determine the resistance offered to the blood, and that in turn is what determines the blood pressure. The vasodilators (literally drugs which widen the blood vessels) cause the blood vessels to relax so that the internal diameter of the vessels widens and this results in a fall in blood pressure. There are many drugs in this group, one of the best being hydralazine (trade name Apresoline).

Hydralazine   The main advantage of hydralazine is that it may be used to supplement other drugs to achieve better control of blood pressure. It can be given on a twice-a-day basis and is quite inexpensive.

Not long after hydralazine was introduced into clinical practice in the early 1950s it fell into disrepute because it was found to cause a rare condition known as the SLE syndrome, which is a generalized disorder affecting the skin, kidneys, blood vessels and joints. However, it is now known that this syndrome occurred because the doses then used were too high, and when the drug was stopped most cases got better spontaneously. We now use lower doses.

Hydralazine also increases the pulse rate, which may be noticeable as palpitation. What happens is that the heart attempts to maintain the pre-existing level of blood pressure by increasing its activity. This is a reflex action and the problem has been solved by giving hydralazine in combination with drugs known to prevent the reflex, such as beta-blockers or methyldopa (see page 96). Today, therefore, hydralazine is not usually used on its own. Other unwanted side-effects include headache and swelling of the ankles.

Prazosin   The trade name for this drug is Hypovase (Minipress in North America and Australia). It acts in a rather similar way to hydralazine, but because its actions are more complex it does not produce the heart reflex associated with hydralazine and other vasodilators. It is a very effective drug and can be used on its own or in combination with other drugs. One important shortcoming, however, is that if the first dose is not sufficiently small an excessive fall in blood pressure may occur; if this happens – and it happens only rarely – the person becomes pale, sweaty and quite distressed. This so-called 'first dose phenomenon' can be avoided by using a very low dose when starting treatment. If there are no symptoms the amount can be increased gradually.

Minoxidil   This is a very new member of the vasodilator group of drugs, and it is not available for clinical use in all countries (its trade name is Loniten). It is a very effective blood-pressure-lowering drug and even the most difficult cases respond to it. However, there are a number of unwanted side-effects, notably fluid retention. It also tends to cause an increase in hair growth. This occurs on the face in particular, but over the rest of the body as well. For these reasons, its use is restricted to those with severe high blood pressure.

Other vasodilators   There are other vasodilators used in the treatment of high blood pressure, but they are usually given only in a hospital setting and to people with very severe high blood pressure. We will not therefore discuss them here.

Drugs acting on the nervous system

How they work
These drugs have in common the ability to get into the nervous system and to interfere with the way in which the brain controls the blood pressure. One group – which includes methyldopa (Aldomet), clonidine (Catapres) and reserpine (Serpasil) – acts in the brain itself, while the remainder – guanethidine (Ismelin) and related drugs – block the sympathetic nervous activity at the level of the nerves themselves. These are the nerves which go to the individual blood vessels.

The group acting on the brain, often called 'centrally acting blood-pressure-lowering drugs', may cause several unwanted side-effects related to the site of action in the brain. To a greater or lesser degree they all can give rise to depression, fatigue, daytime drowsiness, sleep disturbances and dry mouth.

Methyldopa   Methyldopa (trade name Aldomet) has been used for treating high blood pressure for some twenty-five years, and is still widely prescribed. It bears a striking resemblance to adrenaline and probably acts by interfering with the effect of adrenaline. It affects the action of adrenaline in many parts of the body, but most importantly in the brain itself, and blood pressure falls.

With methyldopa the most common problems are depression, tiredness and daytime drowsiness. Less commonly, it may damage the liver and, rarely, cause anaemia. In some people, particularly the elderly, methyldopa causes the blood pressure to fall excessively when the person stands up; when the person is lying down or in a sitting position the blood pressure is quite satisfactory. Doctors call this fall in blood pressure 'postural hypotension'. The problem also occurs, but more commonly, with guanethidine-like drugs.

Methyldopa is often given in four doses every twenty-four hours. We feel that this is probably unnecessary and indeed many doctors now prescribe this drug for use just twice a day. Methyldopa is an effective blood-pressure-lowering drug and many people have taken it for years without apparent ill-effect.

Rauwolfia   The best known drug in this group is reserpine (trade name Serpasil) which, like methyldopa, has been used for over twenty years in the treatment of high blood pressure. Reserpine has its advocates among the more senior physicians who have, as it were, grown up with it. Like methyldopa it lowers blood pressure through its effect on the brain. It can be taken on a once-a-day basis.

Depression is one problem with this drug. This occurs perhaps more frequently and is more severe than with methyldopa and this limits its popularity. However, it is effective as a blood-pressure-lowering drug and can be given on its own.

Clonidine   Clonidine (trade name Catapres) is one of the newer drugs. As with methyldopa and reserpine its main site of action is the brain, where it interferes with the action of adrenaline, thus relaxing the blood vessels in the body.

Many people who take this drug find that at first it causes dry mouth and a feeling of drowsiness during the day. These effects generally wear off after a time, but sometimes they persist and become troublesome.

Clonidine can be used as initial treatment on its own, but more frequently it tends to be prescribed in combination with other drugs for those who are not responding to one drug. It has one serious drawback: if it is stopped abruptly there may be a rebound in blood pressure well above the earlier untreated level. It is very important that anyone taking this drug should know of this possibility. It is a good idea always to have a reserve store of the drug and to be particularly careful that you don't run out of supplies when away from home or on vacation.

Guanethidine (Ismelin) and related drugs   This is a group of drugs which acts on the sympathetic nervous system. They prevent the release of adrenaline from the nerves and thereby allow the blood vessels to relax when they would normally tense up in response to stress and exertion. Unfortunately, we need this mechanism when standing or running. When the system fails the blood goes to the feet and the supply to the brain becomes insufficient, resulting in dizziness or fainting – known as postural hypotension. This is similar to what can happen after standing for a long time in high temperature. Thus the use of these drugs is limited. They were introduced in the early 1960s, but to a large extent have now been superseded by beta-blocking drugs. However, they are still occasionally used, especially for people who have not responded to other drugs. They may also cause diarrhoea, and sometimes impotence in men and failure to ejaculate. Other drugs in this group are bethanidine (trade name Esbatal in Britain and Australia, Esbaloid in Canada) and debrisoquine (trade name Declinax); these are not available in the United States.

The importance of taking your medicine

One all too common reason why high blood pressure fails to respond to treatment is that the person forgets or neglects to take the medicines prescribed. Sometimes the person feels well and fit and therefore sees no reason for continuing with the medicine. Or, conversely, the side-effects may be such that he or she is reluctant to go on with it. From time to time we see patients who stopped treatment when the pills were finished in the mistaken belief that their high blood pressure had been cured; in most cases the high blood pressure cannot be cured as such, but it can be effectively controlled by treatment. However, unless the drugs are taken regularly it will not be possible to control the high blood pressure adequately.

Today there is little excuse for failing to take the drugs you have been prescribed. The availability of relatively non-toxic drugs allows both drug and dose to be tailored to the needs of each individual. Furthermore, it is rarely necessary to have to take the drug more than twice a day.

The precise time of taking the medicine is not important, what is important is that the correct total dose is taken each day. Many people find it useful to link their pill taking with some routine daily activity, brushing their teeth, for example. Some may find it convenient to take their medicine first thing in the morning when they get up and last thing at night when they go to bed. Others may prefer breakfast and evening meal times. Whatever time you choose, it is a good idea to stick to it so that taking your pill becomes an ingrained part of your daily routine.

You must face the fact that if you have high blood pressure

you will probably have to go on taking pills for the rest of your life. On rare occasions it may be possible to stop treatment, but this can only be done safely under the direct supervision of your doctor.

Finally, it is a good idea to keep a record in a notebook of your blood pressure measurements and the drugs you are taking. We supply those attending our blood pressure clinic with a booklet that has one section in which the blood pressure measurement can be entered by doctor, nurse or the patient, and another section for noting down drug treatment. This serves as an excellent means of communication between the patient and the family or hospital doctor. Moreover, if you make a point of always carrying the booklet with you in your wallet or handbag, in the event of an accident the hospital will be aware of the drugs you are taking. You don't need to wait till you are provided with one of these booklets as you can easily make one for yourself along the lines already indicated on page 22.

11 THE FUTURE

Detecting 'hidden' high blood pressure

Over the last thirty years some important advances have been made in our knowledge of high blood pressure: it has been established beyond all doubt that it is a major risk factor in diseases of the heart and circulation; drugs have been developed which effectively lower the blood pressure without causing too many unwanted side-effects; and we now know for sure that if high blood pressure can be brought down to within normal limits, life expectancy will also be brought back to normal. But, as yet, the problem of finding the person who has high blood pressure but no tell-tale symptoms, and whose condition therefore has not been diagnosed, has not been solved.

Much consideration has been given to ways of detecting these people. Perhaps the most logical approach would be to launch a nationwide screening programme, but the cost of this would be enormous, and we do not think it would be justifiable. Modified screening programmes which can be incorporated in existing health clinics may be a compromise. Likewise, the installation of equipment whereby the public can measure their own blood pressure may also be helpful. These machines, if installed in such places as department stores, airports and railway stations, will help a number of people to find out whether they have high blood pressure.

However, in our view the best place for detecting high blood pressure is in the family doctor's office. We know that over a two-year period 80 per cent of the adult population visit their doctor, and if everyone who came had their blood pressure measured, almost all the adult population would be screened every few years.

Improved blood pressure measurement

Despite the technological advances of the last thirty years, there has been remarkably little advance in blood pressure measurement. In fact, if anything, the approach to measurement has become careless and less accurate than it was when the technique was first introduced. Efforts are now being made to influence the medical profession to pay more attention to the details of blood pressure measurement, so that doctors, nurses and medical students are made aware of its limitations as well as its importance The most accurate measurement will be obtained by someone who has been trained in the technique and who uses a mercury sphygmomanometer.

In the future, reliable semi-automated machines may replace the mercury sphygmomanometer, but they will be more expensive. Also, they can only be accepted after reliable and independent centres have assessed the accuracy of their performance over a period of continued use.

Equipment is now being developed that will make it possible to assess the blood pressure response to the stress and activities of daily life over a twenty-four-hour period. Not only will such techniques give greater insight into what exactly constitutes high blood pressure, they will also permit doctors to judge the value and efficacy of their treatment better. However, it must also be recognized that although more and more information will become available, the task of evaluating it all is still a daunting one. Nevertheless, as this approach develops it is likely that people with high blood pressure will be divided into various sub-groups, with perhaps each group needing a different method of treatment.

Pharmacological developments

The most significant step forward in recent years has been the development of beta-blocker drugs, which have made it possible for doctors to prescribe treatment for those people needing drugs without the risk of too many side-effects. Beta-blockers do, however, have their limitations, as we have seen in the previous chapter, and they should be used very cautiously, if at all, on people with asthma and chronic bronchitis.

The vasodilators have also proved to be very effective in the treatment of high blood pressure, but again they are not without side-effects. Improvement in this group of drugs can be expected in the future.

There is a considerable amount of current research into new ways of lowering blood pressure; and a new drug that shows promise is captopril (Capoten – not available in Canada), which interferes with the renin-angiotensin mechanism (see page 16). We can be certain that research into this area will advance considerably in the near future. As research workers study and evaluate mechanisms producing high blood pressure, so they can develop substances that interfere with these mechanisms.

At present the approach to severe high blood pressure is to attack the blood-pressure-controlling system at two or more points. For example, a beta-blocker is given to slow the heart; a diuretic is given to increase the loss of salt and water, and possibly also to widen the blood vessels; the vasodilators are given to reduce the narrowing of the blood vessels; and sometimes a drug which acts on the nervous system, such as methyldopa, is also given. This approach whereby the system is hit at different points means that less of each drug can be used, thus reducing the number of unwanted effects.

Alternative methods

The future also holds promise that other methods of lowering blood pressure, such as biofeedback and transcendental meditation, will be better evaluated and may come to have a place in treatment. If the technique of biofeedback, where the individual is taught to lower his own blood pressure voluntarily, could be standardized and readily applied it might play an important role in the control of high blood pressure.

The need for co-operation with your doctor

One thing that you can do to help improve your outlook for the future is to co-operate with your doctor. That means following his advice about changing your lifestyle and, most important, taking the drugs he prescribes for you. Unfortunately, all too often it happens that someone begins a course of treatment and then drops out for one reason or another. Usually it is because of an unpleasant side-effect, but this is just the time when you should visit your doctor again. Most doctors are very understanding about the problems of long-term drug treatment and will try to find one which suits you. The important thing is to persevere, for in the end it is your life which is at risk.

Conclusions

Whatever advances the future may bring we must return to two fundamental points which, if not acknowledged, will render future developments futile. First, we have to detect those people with high blood pressure – and this can only be done by careful blood pressure measurement of the adult population, and then we must find the most effective way of lowering their blood pressure.

If high blood pressure was effectively reduced, there would be a significant drop in the number of people with cardiovascular disease, especially stroke, and life expectancy would be improved. We know that this is possible and that we have the means to do it.

We believe that if people understand the nature and consequences of high blood pressure, they will make sure that their blood pressure is measured regularly. Furthermore, we hope that a knowledge of blood pressure behaviour will help to establish the co-operation between the medical profession and the public so that high blood pressure can be brought down to within the normal range. It is our hope that this book will contribute towards these goals.

USEFUL ADDRESSES

The following organizations will be able to tell you where to get help:

UNITED STATES

American Heart Association
7320 Greenville Avenue
Dallas
Texas 75231
(or look in your phone book for your local Heart Association)

Citizens for the Treatment of High Blood Pressure (Hypertension)
1101 17th Street N.W.
Suite 608
Washington
DC 20036

Institute of Hypertension Studies
Institute of Hypertension School of Research
7032 Farnsworth
Detroit
Michigan 48211

BRITAIN

British Heart Foundation
57 Gloucester Place
London W1H 4DH
Tel (01) 935 0185

CANADA

Canadian Heart Foundation
1 Nicholas Street
Suite 1200
Ottawa, Ontario
K1N 7B7

Provincial Heart Foundations:

Alberta Heart Foundation
2011 - 10th Avenue S.W.
Calgary, Alberta
T3C OK4
Tel (403) 244 0786

British Columbia Heart Foundation
1212 West Broadway
Vancouver, British Columbia
V6H 3V2
Tel (604) 736 4404

Manitoba Heart Foundation
301 Canada Building
352 Donald Street
Winnipeg, Manitoba
R3B 2H8
Tel (204) 942 0195

New Brunswick Heart Foundation
28 Germain Street
Saint John, New Brunswick
E2L 2E5
Tel (902) 423 7530

Newfoundland Division
Canadian Heart Foundation
152 Water Street
CNT Building
PO Box 5819
St John's, Newfoundland
A1C 5X3
Tel (709) 753 8521

Nova Scotia Heart Foundation
408 Roy Building
1657 Barrington Street
PO Box 1585
Halifax, Nova Scotia
B3J 2Y3
Tel (902) 423 7530

Ontario Heart Foundation
576 Church Street
Toronto, Ontario
M4Y 2S1
Tel (416) 962 3600

Prince Edward Island Division
Canadian Heart Foundation
PO Box 279
51 University Avenue
Charlottetown, PEI
C1A 7K5
Tel (902) 894 8297

Québec Heart Foundation
1455 Peel Street
Suite M-31/32
Montreal, Québec
H3A 1T5
Tel (514) 288 8141

Saskatchewan Heart Foundation
279 - 3rd Avenue North
Saskatoon, Saskatchewan
S7K 2H8
Tel (306) 244 2124

AUSTRALIA

National Heart Foundation of
Australia
55 Townshend Street
Phillip, ACT 2606

NEW ZEALAND

National Heart Foundation of
New Zealand
17 Great South Road
Newmarket
PO Box 17128
Green Lane
Auckland 5
Tel 546 005

IRELAND

Irish Heart Foundation
4 Clyde Road
Ballsbridge
Dublin 4
Tel 685001

SOUTH AFRICA

National Heart Effort
PO Box 70
Tygerberg

ACKNOWLEDGEMENTS

The authors gratefully acknowledge support from the Royal College of Surgeons in Ireland.

The publishers would like to thank the following individuals and organizations for their permission to reproduce illustrative material: A.G.E. Fotostock, Barcelona (page 71); Bavaria Verlag, Munich (frontispiece); John Clutterbuck, New South Wales (page 54); Gruner & Jahr, Munich (page 82); Miller Services, Toronto (page 31); NFB Photothèque, Ottawa (pages 50, 68 and 69); and Adrian Pope, London (cover and pages 23, 24, 26, 27 and 55).

The diagrams on pages 14, 19, 22, 41, 78, 86 and 87 were drawn by David Gifford. The diagram on page 49 was prepared using research material derived from the Canadian Medical Association journal and the World Health Organization.

The cover photograph was modelled by Jenny and Jay Roberts; and the photographs on pages 26 and 27, by Allen Sykes. The table and chair for the photographs on pages 26 and 27 were kindly loaned by William Whitely Ltd, London; and the desk and chairs appearing on the cover were made by Abbess Office Furniture and were kindly loaned by Hill & Noyes Ltd, 23 Bruton Street, London, W1.

Finally, thanks are due to Jennifer Eaton, BSc, MSc, MPS, for information on drug name equivalents and to Dr Patrick Trend for advice in the planning of the step-by-step photography of blood pressure measurement.

INDEX

Other books in the Positive Health Guide series

GET A BETTER NIGHT'S SLEEP
Prof Ian Oswald and Dr Kirstine Adam
For the millions of insomniacs, these world-renowned sleep experts help to break the vicious circle of anxiety over lost sleep leading to more restless nights. They offer practical, scientifically based advice on the best ways to avoid sleeplessness and wake refreshed each morning

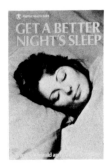

STRESS AND RELAXATION
Self-help ways to cope with stress and relieve nervous tension, ulcers, insomnia, migraine and high blood pressure
Jane Madders
Jane Madders has developed her own simple techniques of natural relaxation that will help to reduce stress in your everyday life. Tension headaches, migraine, insomnia and even nervous breakdown can often be relieved by learning to relax.

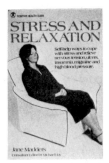

MIGRAINE AND HEADACHES
Understanding, controlling and avoiding the pain
Dr Marcia Wilkinson
In this reassuring guide to coping with one of the commonest and often most distressing medical complaints, Dr Wilkinson explains what makes migraine different from other headaches, how you can identify and avoid the causes of your attacks, and what you can do to deal with the pain. She also gives advice on the action and side-effects of drugs currently used to treat these conditions.

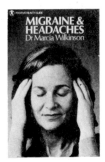

THE BACK – RELIEF FROM PAIN
Patterns of back pain – how to deal with and avoid them
Dr Alan Stoddard

BEAT HEART DISEASE!
A cardiologist explains how you can help your heart and enjoy a healthier life
Prof Risteard Mulcahy

DON'T FORGET FIBRE IN YOUR DIET
To help avoid many of our commonest diseases
Dr Denis Burkitt

ASTHMA AND HAY FEVER
How to relieve wheezing and sneezing
Dr Allan Knight

OVERCOMING ARTHRITIS
A guide to coping with stiff or aching joints
Dr Frank Dudley Hart

PSORIASIS
A guide to one of the commonest skin diseases
Prof Ronald Marks

DIABETES
A practical new guide to healthy living
Dr Jim Anderson

THE DIABETICS' DIET BOOK
A new high-fibre eating programme
Dr Jim Mann and the Oxford Dietetic Group

THE HIGH-FIBRE COOKBOOK
Recipes for good health
Pamela Westland
Introduced by Dr Denis Burkitt

VARICOSE VEINS
How they are treated, and what you can do to help
Prof Harold Ellis

ECZEMA AND DERMATITIS
How to cope with inflamed skin
Prof Rona MacKie

ENJOY SEX IN THE MIDDLE YEARS
Dr Christine Sandford